Wells'

Supportive Therapies in Health Care

Edited by Richard Wells
and Verena Tschudin

Baillière Tindall

LONDON • PHILADELPHIA • SYDNEY • TOKYO • TORONTO

Baillière Tindall
W. B. Saunders

24–28 Oval Road
London NW1 7DX

The Curtis Center
Independence Square West
Philadelphia, PA 19106-3399, USA

Harcourt Brace & Company
55 Horner Avenue
Toronto, Ontario, M8Z 4X6, Canada

Harcourt Brace & Company, Australia
30–52 Smidmore Street
Marrickville
NSW 2204, Australia

Harcourt Brace & Company (Japan) Inc
Ichibancho Central Building
22-1 Ichibancho
Chiyoda-ku, Tokyo 102, Japan

A catalogue record for this book is available from the British Library

ISBN 0–7020–1591–1

Typeset by Columns Design and Production Services Ltd, Reading, Berkshire
Printed and bound in Great Britain by Butler and Tanner Ltd, Frome, Somerset

RM 700 e

Wells'

Supportive
Therapies in
Health Care

Contents

There is a colour plate section between pages 46 and 47

Contributors

Sheila Conachy
Sister, Raven Ward, Rehabilitation Unit, The Royal Marsden Hospital, Fulham Road, London SW3 6JJ

Camilla Connell
Art Therapist, The Royal Marsden Hospital, Fulham Road, London SW3 6JJ

Maureen Hunter
Rehabilitation Services Manager, The Royal Marsden Hospital, Fulham Road, London SW3 6JJ

Sheena Hildebrand
Therapeutic Masseuse, Rehabilitation Department, The Royal Marsden Hospital, Downs Road, Sutton, Surrey SM2 5PT

Chris Jarmey
European Shiatsu School, Central Administration, High Banks, Lockeridge, Nr Marlborough, Wiltshire SN8 4EQ

Anne Lett
British School – Reflex Zone Therapy of the Feet, Oakington Avenue, Wembley Park, London HA9 8HY

Jane Mallett
Research Co-ordinator, The Royal Marsden Hospital, Fulham Road, London SW3 6JJ

Ray Rowden
Director, Institute of Health Services Management, Chalton Street, London NW1 7JD

Lynne Ryman
Sister, Radiotherapy Department, The Royal Marsden Hospital, Fulham Road, London SW3 6JJ

Geoffrey Wadlow
Co-Principal, London School of Acupuncture and Traditional Chinese Medicine, Bunhill Row, London EC1

Regan C. Wright
Head Art Therapist, St Bernards Psychiatric Wing, Ealing Hospital, Uxbridge Road, Southall, Middlesex

Verena Tschudin
Counsellor and Writer; Honorary Lecturer, University of East London, Romford Road, London E15 4LZ

Foreword

This publication is a welcome addition to the growing library of material on supportive therapies and the way in which they are now beginning to be recognised in their own right. The previous decade has seen a remarkable expansion of professional attitudes and public requirements for health care. The underlying causes for these changes are not immediately clear, but certain events have acted as decisive signals.

Perhaps two of the most significant can be associated with HRH The Prince of Wales. His perception during his year as President of the British Medical Association in 1982 led to a speech in which he sought to redefine the principles of medical treatment in the light of traditional thinking of the middle ages. A decade later Prince Charles again reflected the progress which has been made in the understanding of complementary medicine. In a message of encouragement to an ICM Conference in September 1993 in London, the Prince suggested that the time had come for complementary medicine, and for such conferences to be seen as a further sign of its steady assimilation into the wider framework of health care in this country.

Prince Charles suggested that the best of conventional, clinical medicine combined with the best of complementary therapies and co-ordinated via enlightened, better-educated doctors and primary-care professionals was the way forward. He expected the rewards to be immense: the reduction of dependence, and expense, on drugs; and a sympathetic broadening of the options we can offer the afflicted. Once again Prince Charles encapsulated the thoughts and aspirations of most people in health care. But the position today has not come about without exhaustive and painstaking efforts by such people as Richard Wells.

So often one hears the remark that 'there is no scientific evidence to suggest . . .' Such a statement is capable of two meanings. The first might indicate that investigations have been completed without any significant result being obtained, whilst the second might suggest that no tests have been made at all. Scientists tell us that research must be carried out using the double-blind trial. However, this method assumes that every person has the same problems and there are similar causative factors. Whilst this can be helpful for the symptomatic approach to diagnosis and treatment, it is not appropriate to the traditional methods of health care which require more information. These approaches have an additional element in the diagnosis known as the vitality, energy field or spirit. The precise description changes with the system, for example, in Chinese Medicine the energy is called *Qi*; in Homoeopathy it is vitality; in Healing it is spirit, and so on. These systems suggest that disease comes about when the relationship between the physical body, mind and vitality (spirit) are not correctly functioning in relation to each other. This is known as lack of balance and the complementary practitioner will seek to ensure that a correct balance is restored.

The extent of the patient's problem lies in the cause of these imbalances and the time taken to bring about change. The most important decision has to be to decide at which level the imbalance is seated – is it purely physical, purely mental and emotional or at vitality level? Is it a combination of all? For the complementary practitioner, these factors must be determined before treatment can begin.

The symptomatic diagnosis can be a useful pointer but it is not always complete and it can be fascinating to watch complementary practitioners at work. The length and complexity of the homoeopathic diagnosis is well known, with many questions being asked about seemingly unimportant and unconnected factors. In the same way, the Chinese can obtain information from six different pulse points on each wrist whilst others simply count the heartbeats.

A further factor which is common to all complementary methods is the commitment of the patients to take part in their own healing. This requires discussion between the patient and practitioner in addition to the actual physical therapy. This communication can be used to encourage the patient to learn to relax and to begin to understand how to take control of life, interpersonal relationships, nutrition, the environment and all the other factors which can cause anxiety, tension and subsequent disease.

In spite of many difficulties, research is going forward with more emphasis on the audit method of assessment. The anecdotal evidence, which is so obvious to those immediately concerned, is now being assessed as part of a co-ordinated programme and we expect some useful input over the next 5-year period.

Perhaps the most important and difficult aspect has been the work to establish standards of education. Hundreds of courses are regularly advertised but there is no national standard of training. The casual enquirer therefore has no means of knowing the value of the course offered. A brand name such as Reflexology can be used with varying levels of competence and the patient needs to know the extent of the practitioner's skill. Some idea of the problem can be seen from the example of aromatherapy. A practitioner can be called an Aromatherapist after studying a few oils and can use it for relaxation in an hairdressing salon. A beautician can use the title Aromatherapist after studying about 35 to 40 oils but will also know some differential diagnosis and be able to recognise some contra-indications. More expert practitioners will have studied and be able to use over 160 oils and have a greater understanding of both the patient's physiology and the treatment potential. At present all can use the same title.

The public has little means of assessing the difference. Most registers of practitioners have no statutory status and many are simply an in-house listing of members. A similar situation existed for teaching bodies, schools and colleges which can issue their own certificates or diplomas without being required to have any external examiners or reference to any outside regulatory body. However, this position will change in the near future with the introduction of National Vocational Qualifications (NVQs) and the formal accreditation of many courses in complementary medicine.

The introduction of the concept of NVQs has caused considerable problems, not least because of so many different approaches to the same subject. In 1987, there were over 80 diplomas and certificates being offered in hypnotherapy alone. Training varied from one weekend to two years. Similar problems existed in other disciplines. The complementary movement has been divided in its attitude to NVQs. In general, the teaching bodies which have prided themselves on offering a professional training have welcomed them as a means of additional confirmation of standards. However, some Registers have been more cautious or simply ignored them altogether.

In September 1993, the Institute for Complementary Medicine had over 300 affiliated organisations working towards accreditation and NVQs. The numbers are still growing. The British Register of Complementary Practitioners has 18 Divisions with each representing a discipline or therapy. Another development is the International College of Complementary Medicine which will provide a focal point for training in most disciplines and help to co-ordinate a world-wide approach. The Royal College of Nursing and the Institute of Advanced Nursing Education have introduced modules in aromatherapy, hypnotherapy and massage as part of the Advanced Nursing Degree. Reflexology is part of another programme of nurse education in the process of accreditation. There are a number of other umbrella organisations and councils attempting to achieve accreditation and still more registers and groupings being formed – the array is bewildering to the onlooker.

Supportive Therapies in Health Care brings together a number of approaches to patient care which have been steadily gaining public and media interest since the 1960s. This is the period which is generally thought of as the beginning of the complementary approach to cancer care in the multi-discipline format. I remember this because my father died of cancer at that time when I began my own quest for ways in which to add to the conventional treatments. Working in the hospital was both a privilege and a challenge at a time when healing and visualisation techniques were considered well-meaning but ineffectual. When patients did make unexpected progress with these treatments or simply said they felt better, it was usually put down to either a wrong medical diagnosis in the first place, spontaneous remission, or imagination. The problem for the practitioner was always keeping a balance between maintaining a positive outlook for the patient and giving an unreasonable expectation of a cure.

The importance of the work of Richard Wells and those who shared his belief cannot be understated. If a patient feels better for whatever reason and there are no toxic side-effects, then the patient should have the right to get the help. The fact that the reasons why this help lifts the patient's spirits are not fully understood is no argument for not providing it.

The chapters cover a variety of therapeutic approaches and each author provides a comprehensive survey of their understanding.

Maureen Hunter, writing on nutritional therapies, quotes Hutchinson and Mottram (1933) who suggested that 'In the matter of diet every man must, in the last resort, be law unto himself . . .' This is especially important because the causes of illness vary from patient to patient even when similar symptoms are present. The fact that this nutritional fact was understood as long ago as 1933 is yet another example of an 'idea whose time has come'. It also restates the principles of all aspects of complementary medicine. Ms Hunter concludes that sound balanced information and advice should be sought from a registered practitioner. Whilst this is good advice, it is also true that practitioners are frequently required to accept new ideas which appear to have scientific merit but which are later contradicted by other research.

To the patient there is much contradictory information appearing from different scientific sources. A decade ago the idea that nutrition could have an effect on a child's behaviour and intellectual capacity was considered laughable, and yet tests have since suggested otherwise. The behaviour of prisoners appeared to be affected by diet. Precisely why these results were obtained and whether they are repeatable remains to be seen. This is the argument for correctly designed research protocols which take all matters of human consciousness into consideration. It shows the enormous breadth of scope and understanding required to recognise the full potential of nutritional treatment. The same arguments can be put forward for all areas of complementary treatment. It further confirms the need for specific diagnosis related to individual needs rather than the broad treatment regimens or diets which are so common in the media.

Aromatherapy, Reflexology (Reflex Zone Therapy), Acupuncture and Shiatsu are described in a supportive role, but it should be remembered that each has much to offer as a full treatment regimen in its own right. Geoffrey Wadlow correctly highlights the fact that acupuncture is often restricted to pain control, but Chinese Medicine brings 4000 years of knowledge and experience to all health matters. The other disciplines have similar historical backgrounds waiting to be re-discovered.

Perhaps the most revealing chapters are those discussing relaxation and visualisation, music, sound, art and laughter. All these are often thought of as part of everyday life (or should be) and yet are described here in terms of their therapeutic value.

Meditation has always been a central pillar of religious life since it involves the act of linking the physical, mental, emotional and spiritual aspects of consciousness. The 1960s were notable for many innovations such as video recording, colour television, the Beatles and the Maharishi. Once the Beatles had taken to transcendental meditation, the whole process of mind control became more widely attractive, with different methods suddenly competing for converts. This time also saw the beginning of the use of relaxation and visualisation in the treatment of cancer and by the early 1970s case histories were being published by Carl and Stephanie Simonton which described their work in these areas. It was during this period also that the effectiveness of music and laughter became more widely understood. The harmonic variations of some music can be especially useful in bringing deep relaxation and emotional release. Laughter has always been considered the 'best medicine'.

The publishers have brought together writers who have provided an excellent background to each of their subjects. The development of these approaches to health care will bring about a gradual appreciation of the underlying principles and the subtle energies which are involved at all levels of human consciousness.

In the final analysis all healing must be based on truth. The search for truth and the inner compassion which unites all practitioners, irrespective of race, creed, colour or political affiliation, will drive forward research and development so that all may receive the best treatment for their condition at any time. Each patient will also be encouraged to play a part in their treatment which must be based on adequate information and personal choice.

Richard Wells was primarily concerned with cancer but both he and his co-editor, Verena Tschudin, are to be congratulated because this book will also have a significance for all those concerned with chronic conditions. One feels that they would have had particular sympathy with the words of Paracelsus, 'Would we humans knew our hearts in truth nothing would be impossible for us.'

MICHAEL ENDACOTT
Deputy Director
Institute for Complementary Medicine
September 1993

Preface

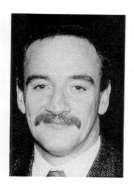

Every author has a story to tell about his or her book. This book has a very particular story – not least because its key author is – tragically – no longer here to tell it. So it falls to me to tell it, and I consider that to be a special privilege.

When Richard Wells took up the position of Rehabilitation Services Manager at the Royal Marsden Hospital in London, everyone involved knew that this would be a venture with a difference. Richard had a vision of what care could be like and seemingly turned this into reality overnight. Since he never settled for anything second-best or half-finished, he managed to pull a team together who shared his enthusiasm. Into this remit came a whole array of complementary – or supportive – therapies which were not usually on hospital lists of treatments or therapies offered. Richard naturally cared holistically for patients, which meant their families, partners and friends were included in this care. He knew that patients worry about their close ones, and that they can be severely affected by the 'patient's' state of health. By including complementary therapies in his care, this meant that close ones could be more easily involved in the care, taking part with the patient in these therapies, and receiving them themselves at the same time, if they wanted to. Richard believed that complementary therapies did not necessarily need validating by science or medicine: if a patient said that he or she *felt better* for it, then this was his justification for providing it – with or without the backup of research. It semed to be natural then that Richard should bring these therapies together in a book, to give other health care professionals an incentive to introduce them also in their settings.

This book stresses the 'supportive' aspects of these therapies. In this setting this is perhaps a truer term to use than 'complementary' or 'alternative'. The book does not intend to cover the full range of complementary therapies, nor is it meant to be a text on 'how to do' the therapies. Seeing these therapies as *supportive* suggests that they can be widely used. Because of this the book does not validate any of the courses or addresses mentioned in the Appendix; names and addresses are given simply so that those interested in any subject might have a starting-point for further research.

The increasing trend among health care professionals, especially nurses, to turn to supportive therapies is, however, furthered by this book. Many of the authors in this book were chosen from among the therapists active around Richard. But they all stress that the therapies they describe in use with cancer patients are not limited to that group of patients.

Towards the end of the writing of the chapters it became clear that Richard would not be able to continue as editor, and that is when he invited me to take on the role of co-editor.

The book was originally planned to contain a few more therapies than the ones presented here. The intention is now to make the book not only a memorial, but a *living* memorial, to Richard and his work, in that future editions are envisaged with more therapies included as they become more known, more available and more acceptable in patient care. The publishers would appreciate suggestions and ideas for chapters and authors from the readers and in this way this will be a truly 'supportive' book.

Verena Tschudin

Acknowledgements

The publisher wishes to thank the following for the use of their illustrations, whose copyright they remain:

The Royal Marsden Hospital – colour plates 3.1–3.13
Hanne Marquardt – colour plate 9.1
Ray Rowden – Figures in Chapter 2
Chris Jarmey and Gabriel Mojay – Figures in Chapter 7

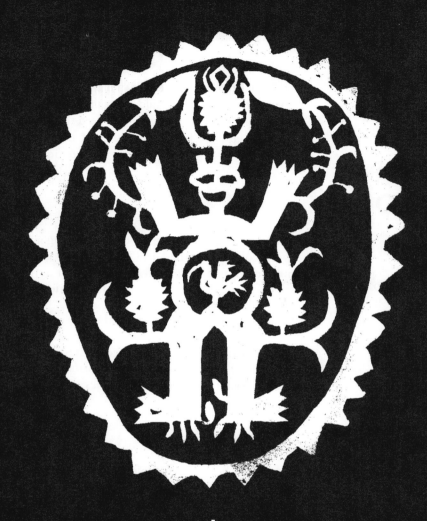

I
NUTRITIONAL THERAPY

Maureen Hunter

In the matter of diet every man must, in the last resort, be a law
unto himself; but he should draw up his dietetic code intelligently,
and apply it honestly, giving due heed to the warnings which Nature
is sure to address to him should he at any time transgress.

Hutchinson and Mottram 1933[1]

Definitions

Nutrition is defined as the process of feeding and of being nourished.
The word comes from the Latin 'nutritio' and the French 'nourir', both
meaning to nourish. In animals the process of nutrition involves the
ingestion, digestion, absorption and assimilation of nutrients present in
the diet.

Nutritional therapy can be defined as the study of the interactions of
nutritional factors with human physiology and biochemistry. The
clinical application of the knowledge of these interactions in the
maintenance of health and in the prevention and treatment of disease
forms the basis of the science of *dietetics*.

History

Since the earliest times people have been preoccupied with the
relationship between food and health. Nutrition as a science is said to
have been founded by Lavoisier towards the end of the eighteenth
century, but dietetics is a much older subject. In the days of ancient
Greece, Hippocrates frequently gave his patients advice about what
foods they should eat. In the Eastern world, Oriental medicine has been
using diet and changes in diet as a major therapy in the treatment of
ailments and diseases for thousands of years. Only over the past 20
years has the science of nutrition developed sufficiently to allow
quantative recommendations to be made about the amount and type of
food which should be eaten to maintain health.

During the first forty years of this century major advances in nutrition
were made as diseases which had long been familiar became identified
with deficiencies of single nutrients that were essential in only small
amounts. The often dramatic improvement resulting from the
administration of a food known to contain the nutrient, and later of the
nutrient itself, captured the interest of doctors and scientists alike. The
discovery of these substances, named vitamins, marked the beginning of
a major chapter in nutritional history.

Nutrition and dietetics are, like all scientific disciplines, ever expanding and constantly developing. As they do so we see the major role that nutrition and nutrition advice has in the maintenance of health and in the treatment of disease. Yet, until recently, nutrition has not been given a high priority in our health-care system or in our educational system. Dietitians, nutritionists and other health-care workers with an interest in nutrition have been campaigning for many years now to have nutrition recognised as a major factor in health care. In 1981 Professor Yudkin, Professor of Nutrition at the University of London, expressed the importance of nutrition as follows:

> I make no apology for saying that the health of the majority of human beings depends more on their nutrition than it does on any other single factor. However important and dramatic have been the advances in hygiene, medicine and surgery, it is still true that even more important will be the effects proper nutrition would have on human morbidity and mortality. For this reason, I believe that the ultimate objective of nutritionists must be the nutrition education of the public. [2]

The science of nutrition and dietetics has evolved so much in the last two or three decades that it is now studied and practised as a discipline and profession separate from, but complementary to, the medical and nursing professions.

The State Registered Dietitian undergoes four years of specialist academic and clinical training in the science of nutrition, physiology, biochemistry and other related topics. Most dietitians and all newly qualified dietitians hold university degrees and all are state registered.

The role of the dietitian is varied, and he or she may practise in areas such as health education and disease prevention, therapeutic diets and clinical practice, food science, the food industry and education and research.

In January 1992, The King's Fund published a report entitled *A Positive Approach to Nutrition as Treatment*.[3] It states that many people with severe illness are at risk from malnutrition which often goes unrecognised, and claims that doctors and nurses frequently fail to recognise under-nourishment because they are not trained to look for it. The report investigates the clinical and financial benefits of nutritional treatment of the malnourished patient and sets out aims and recommendations for the future.

However, it is not just in the areas of malnutrition or severe illness that nutritional or dietary therapy is of major importance. It is now widely known and accepted that nutrition plays a major role in the aetiology and treatment of many diseases. Examples of these in developed countries include heart disease, obesity, diabetes, cancer, coeliac disease and so on. In developing countries examples include protein-energy malnutrition, rickets and beriberi.

On the other hand, the use of nutrition and nutritional therapy as part of homoeopathic, holistic and complementary regimes has become increasingly popular and has received much media coverage in recent years. This has been received with mixed feelings and scepticism by conventional nutritionists and dietitians, as much of the dietary advice given in these circumstances appears to have no proven mode of action, though many patients perceive benefits. Health foods and health-food stores, unheard of ten years ago, are now found on almost every high street. Their use is becoming increasingly popular and fashionable. There is a wealth of products and literature available, but the products vary widely in terms of claims and actual benefit and the reliability of the nutritional information published is often questionable.

There are a number of regulatory bodies and organisations whose role it is to monitor and regulate the practice of nutritional or dietary therapy. Firstly, the Council for Professions Supplementary to Medicine control the state registration of appropriately trained dietitians. It is impossible to work in the NHS as a dietitian without this registration. Unfortunately, any persons, qualified or not, can call themselves a 'nutritionist' or 'dietitian' and set up practice outside the NHS. This has led to many problems, especially in the area of alternative or complementary medicine. A register is now being compiled of all appropriately qualified nutritionists and dietitians so that health-care professionals and the public will be able to check the therapists' credibility before seeking advice. Other organisations involved in the research and practice of nutritional and dietary therapy include the British Dietetic Association and the British Nutrition Foundation. A list of these organisations can be found at the end of this chapter.

This chapter sets out to examine the role of nutrition as a supportive therapy in health care today.

Mode
of action

Nutritional therapy or dietary therapy can be said to work in a number of different ways. The basic action of nutritional therapy is to provide an adequate intake of the energy and nutrients required by the body, in the best way possible, either to maintain or restore optimum health or to treat disease.

The body needs energy to perform mechanical work, to maintain the tissues of the body and for growth. Most of the energy in food is ultimately converted to heat and its dissipation maintains the body temperature. At the most, a person can convert 25 per cent of the energy in food into mechanical work. Of the energy required for maintenance, less than 10 per cent is used for internal mechanical work; for example, the beating of the heart or the movement of respiratory muscles. Over 90 per cent is used for the synthesis of protein and other macromolecules.[4]

The nutrients which the body requires are:

- carbohydrates as a source of energy;
- protein for the growth and repair of tissue;
- fat as a source of energy, vitamins and essential fatty acids;
- vitamins for metabolic processes;
- minerals for metabolic processes, skeletal growth and muscle action;
- water for the regulation of cell water and fluid balance.

Specific nutritional therapies have specific modes of action, and these are too numerous and too complex to allow discussion in this chapter. The mode of action of the major types of therapies which are proven and well researched are discussed later.

There are nutritional therapies in use, as stated above, that have no scientifically proven mode of action. These include macrobiotics, raw food diets, cleansing diets, fad reducing diets and food-combining diets.

Macrobiotics is an Oriental way of eating based on the 'yin–yang' theory. Yin and yang represent the opposing forces in life, and these must be kept in balance for optimum spiritual and physical health. Foods are classified into yin and yang according to where and how they are grown or produced. The theory states that when foods which are at the extremes of yin and yang comprise the mainstay of the diet for any length of time, the physiological condition becomes imbalanced and this leads to disease. The macrobiotic dietary approach is not a specifically defined diet since the basic philosophy states that all individuals are different and therefore individual diets differ according to state of health and presence of disease.

Raw food diets claim many benefits but have no particular theory of action.

Cleansing diets claim in theory to be able to remove the 'toxins' from the modern diet and relieve such ailments as arthritis and catarrh.

Fad reducing diets claim in theory to work by 'speeding up metabolism' or by 'burning up fat' more effectively than any other type of weight-reducing diet.

Food-combining diets claim that some modern degenerative diseases are the result of eating the wrong combination of foods; for example, protein-containing and carbohydrate-containing foods at the same meal. Various rules are laid down governing the types of foods which may be eaten at any one time.

Another type of nutritional therapy is one sometimes referred to as 'nutritional medicine'. In this type of therapy, individual nutrients or foods or combinations of nutrients or foods are used in a therapeutic manner rather like a drug therapy, in order to cure or treat a specific disease or disorder.

Benefits

The benefits of a nutritional therapy can broadly be described as physiological and/or psychological and can be divided into the following categories:

- the maintenance of health;
- the treatment of primary nutritional disorders;
- the treatment of other disorders and diseases.

THE MAINTENANCE OF HEALTH

Good health depends on many factors – food, heredity, climate, hygiene, exercise – but food is the most important of all these. Provision of a nutritionally adequate and hygienic diet, in a socially equitable fashion, confers major health benefits, including:

- elimination of dietary deficiency diseases;
- reduction of acute and chronic food-borne diseases;
- improvements in overall nutritional status, including increased childhood growth rates;
- increased resistance to bacterial and parasitic infectious diseases.

A major consequence of the increase in knowledge and practice of good nutrition has been an increase in life expectancy. However, in affluent societies, the problem of diet-related chronic disease has become apparent over recent decades. These chronic diseases are, in part, manifestations of nutrient excesses and imbalances in the 'Western affluent' diet, so they are in principle largely preventable. Examples include, particularly, coronary heart disease, cerebrovascular disease, various cancers, diabetes mellitus, gallstones, dental caries, gastro-intestinal disorders, and various bone and joint diseases.[5] The enormous cost of the high-technology, tertiary health care needed for the diagnosis and management of these high-incidence chronic diseases is already apparent. The benefits of reducing the future burdens of these diseases are obvious, and action to prevent or reduce their incidence is both a social responsibility and an economic necessity.

One major source of action is change of diet. The diet of affluence is characterised by an excess of energy-dense foods rich in fat and sugars but low in complex carbohydrates (the main source of dietary fibre). Epidemiological research has demonstrated a close and consistent link between this type of diet and the emergence of the diseases listed above. Scientific evidence continues to accumulate supporting this relationship.[6] Excess intake of saturated fats and elevated levels of blood cholesterol are linked with coronary heart disease. The main risk factor for strokes is high blood pressure, in which obesity, alcohol intake and excess salt intake play major contributory roles. Obesity is strongly related to the development of diabetes. It has been estimated that approximately one-third of cancers are associated with dietary factors. For example, an excess of dietary fat has been linked to an increased risk of cancers of the breast and colon. The role of nutritional therapy in the prevention of disease is an area now receiving much attention, and the education of the population in the principles of healthy eating is of major importance.

THE TREATMENT OF PRIMARY NUTRITIONAL DISORDERS

Primary nutritional disorders are those where an aspect of diet is the major cause of the disease or disorder and where nutritional therapy is, therefore, a vital treatment. Many of these disorders are associated with an inadequate food intake and include starvation, protein-energy malnutrition, endemic goitre, xerophthalmia, rickets and osteomalacia, pellagra and scurvy. These diseases are almost unheard of in the Western world but are extremely common in the developing countries, where droughts, food shortages and famine are everyday problems. In these circumstances it is the poor, expectant mothers, children and the elderly who are most at risk. These diseases are still present on a scale that would horrify us all, and recent television coverage of famines has highlighted the scale of the problem which faces the world. Each year millions of young children die of protein-energy malnutrition, hundreds of thousands become permanently blind due to vitamin A deficiency and tens of thousands are born only to become cretinous deaf-mutes due to iodine deficiency. In the countries of the Third World, birth rate exceeds death rate and the population is expanding, whereas in the Western world the population growth is declining. This, combined with droughts, crop failure, natural disaster, war, political and economic factors, leads to low standards of nutrition and the onset of disastrous famines.

The benefits of the knowledge and practice of nutritional therapy in these situations lies in the development of nutrition policies and educational programmes relevant to the rural population in these countries. They mainly take the form of applied nutrition programmes which are made up of interrelated educational activities aimed at the improvement of local food production, consumption and distribution in favour of local communities, particularly mothers and children in rural areas. These are usually co-ordinated by the international relief agencies who also have a role in surveillance so as to give early warning of impending famine.

Not all the primary nutritional disorders are confined to the developing world. Two major disorders found in Western countries are obesity and anorexia nervosa. Obesity, the most prevalent nutritional disorder in prosperous communities, is the result of an incorrect energy balance leading to an increased store of energy, mainly as fat. It is, in general, a preventable disorder. Obesity increases the risk of developing many diseases and is a disorder that should be taken seriously. When obesity is severe, one or more of these diseases is likely to impair health, and life expectancy is greatly reduced. Nutritional therapy is simple in principle, though not always in practice. Slimming has become big business, and books and articles on slimming diets abound. Much of the information is misleading and some is false and dangerous. Because of this, many people become confused about nutritional therapy and weight loss. Obesity is an inevitable result of eating more than is needed, and the only way to slim is to reduce the amount of food eaten. The benefits to the patient are those of better general health, reduced risk of further obesity-related diseases such as heart disease and an improvement in body image and general quality of life. Such people then become less of a burden to the community and to the health-care system.

Anorexia nervosa is a psychiatric disorder arising from, or resulting in, a refusal to eat, which often leads to severe emaciation. Since about 1970 it has become more prevalent and mainly affects adolescent girls and young women, but cases are seen in older women and in men. The central abnormality is a desire to obtain and then maintain a low body weight. The primary aim of nutritional therapy is to get the patient to eat in order to restore nutritional status. In many patients the benefits of nutritional therapy are short-lived as they often continue, or return to, dietary restrictions.

THE TREATMENT OF OTHER DISEASES AND DISORDERS

A number of diseases, many of which are common and well known, involve nutritional therapy as part of their management, because modification of the usual diet or the provision of a special diet reduces the metabolic burden on disordered organs or relieves symptoms and other manifestations of the disease. It is not the intention of this chapter to discuss detailed therapeutic dietetics but to give an overview of the role nutritional therapy plays and the benefits it can impart to the patient. The table below highlights the major disorders and diseases where nutritional therapy has important benefits. In each of the conditions the effects of the disorder may be neutralised, or the functional state of an organ and the patient's health improved, by the nature of the diet.

Disease/disorder	Nutritional/dietary therapy
Phenylketonuria	low phenylalanine
Galactosaemia	milk free
Lactose intolerance	lactose free
Coeliac disease	gluten free
Food allergy	elimination of allergenic food
Renal failure	low protein
Nephrotic syndrome	high protein
Diabetes mellitus	low sugar
Pancreatic disease	low fat
Weight loss and malnutrition	high energy, high protein
Dysphagia	texture modification
Nausea	light diet, low fat
Bowel disorders	modification of fibre
Hyperlipidaemias	modification of fat

Medical and nutritional science has provided a firm scientific basis for the above aspects of nutritional therapy. There are, however, nutritional therapies in use which have little, if any, scientific validity. It is easy and tempting to reject such therapies but some people do seem to find them beneficial. Macrobiotic and some homoeopathic therapies are included in this category. Due to their lack of scientific validity, most conventional nutritionists and dietitians are reluctant to recommend them or accept their use. For any nutritional therapy to be accepted, the benefits it imparts for the patient must outweigh any associated harm, and following the therapy must not put the patient's overall nutritional status at risk, or cause it to deteriorate. Unfortunately, many of the unproven nutritional therapies used, especially those advocated for life-threatening diseases such as cancer or AIDS, do have more risk of harm than benefits and can contribute towards a deterioration in nutritional status. This is what makes it difficult for recognised nutritional experts to accept their use or for reliable clinical trials to be carried out. This means that these regimes tend to be recommended and publicised by 'alternative practitioners' and non-scientific publications. However, medicine is an art as well as a science, and some unproven nutritional therapies do seem to have some benefit, so we must keep an open mind as to their use in the treatment of some disorders. It must be stated, though, that the benefit imparted by such therapies is likely to be one of increased well-being, and possibly symptom control, rather than any specific physiological or medical one.[7] An increase in well-being is an important aspect of feeling better and we must be careful not to underestimate its importance in health care. Providing that the increase in well-being is not at the expense of a poor nutritional status, such nutritional therapies should be taken seriously. Some of the conditions for which unproven nutritional therapies are often advocated are listed below:

Gastrointestinal conditions; e.g. irritable bowel syndrome, inflammatory bowel disease, flatulence
Cancer
AIDS
Arthritis
Bronchitis
Emphysema
Asthma
Hay fever
Cystitis

Kidney stones
Eczema and dermatitis
Menstrual problems
Infertility
Preconceptional care
Infections
Candidiasis
Disorders of the nervous system
Migraine and related headaches
Hyperactivity
Food allergy

Applications

The application of the theory of nutritional therapy to everyday practice can be split into the following areas:

* healthy eating and nutrition education;
* nutritional support;
* therapeutic dietetics;
* unproven or complementary dietary therapies.

HEALTHY EATING AND NUTRITION EDUCATION

In order to reduce the risk of diet-related diseases, the goal of nutritional therapy must be to moderate or remove the excesses in the present diet that contribute to the high incidence of these diseases. There are two main sets of guidelines to help achieve these goals in practice. The first are the official recommended daily amounts of certain nutrients for different age groups and sexes. Every country has its own figures, and the UK recommendations by the Department of Health can be found in the book *Dietary Reference Values for Food Energy and Nutrients for the United Kingdom*.[8]

The second set of guidelines comes from the various reports produced by groups of nutritional experts. These reports give recommendations on specific aspects of diet and often describe how dietary changes can be achieved. The most important report of the 1980s was the NACNE report.[9] This report proposed nutritional guidelines for health education in Britain. Another significant report was one on diet and cardiovascular disease, known as the COMA report, which was produced by the DHSS in 1984.[10] The most recent report on diet, nutrition and health was produced by the British Medical Association in 1986. Fortunately, doctors, dietitians and others involved in health education are in agreement about what constitutes a healthy diet, the principles of which are described below:

- eat a wide variety of foods;
- maintain a healthy weight;
- eat plenty of high fibre foods;
- reduce fat intake;
- reduce sugar intake;
- eat plenty of fruit and vegetables;
- drink alcohol in sensible amounts.

The role of the dietitian, and others involved in nutrition education is to help individuals translate these guidelines into practical hints for everyday eating.

NUTRITIONAL SUPPORT

Ill persons, whether in hospital or not, are at risk of malnutrition once they become unable to consume an adequate nutritional intake. The resulting deterioration in nutritional status seriously delays recovery from medical and surgical disorders, and at worst is life-threatening. The reasons for a reduction in food intake in illness are many and varied, and include:

- chronic pain;
- depression and anxiety;
- physical handicap affecting ability to prepare or eat food;
- difficulty in chewing or swallowing;
- nausea and vomiting;
- general loss of appetite;
- diarrhoea;
- constipation.

In these circumstances, the role of nutritional therapy is to provide adequate nutritional support in order to prevent malnutrition occurring or to treat it if it is already present. Good, regular nutritional assessment of patients in hospital is vital in order to recognise the onset of nutritional problems and to take appropriate action to alleviate them. Any patient who is at risk of becoming, or who has already become, malnourished should be referred to a dietitian or nutrition team for expert assessment and advice.

Nutritional support can either be provided by the enteral route, which includes oral feeding and tube feeding, or the parenteral route – that is, intravenous feeding. Enteral feeding would always be the method of choice and parenteral feeding should only be considered if the function of the gastro-intestinal tract is impaired.

The simplest way to provide nutritional support is to help the patient to eat more. This can be achieved by the use of small, frequent meals or snacks of appetising or favourite foods. If this method fails to provide an adequate nutritional intake, then the use of commercially available nutritional supplements may be recommended. These are available in different forms, such as drinks or powders, and can be used as well as, or instead of, normal foods to increase a patient's nutritional intake.

If the above methods fail to provide an adequate intake or if the patient is unable to take any food orally, then it will be necessary to use artificial nutritional support in the form of tube feeding. A wide range of commercially available, nutritionally complete enteral feeds are available which can be administered via a choice of routes. These are

- nasogastric;
- nasoduodenal;
- nasojejunal;
- gastrostomy (feeding tube place directly into the stomach via the abdominal wall);
- jejunostomy (feeding tube surgically inserted directly into the jejunum via the abdominal wall);
- oesophagostomy (feeding tube placed into the oesophagus via the side of the neck).

In all the above cases the use of fine-bore feeding tubes is recommended. Tube feeding is inexpensive, relatively free of complications and is usually well tolerated by patients.

The use of parenteral feeding – the infusion of nutrients in special solutions into a vein – should only be undertaken when it is impossible to maintain an adequate nutritional intake using the gastro-intestinal tract. Parenteral nutrition is expensive and can lead to metabolic and infective complications.

In order for any method of nutritional support to be effective there must be good liaison and teamwork between doctors, dietitians, nurses and caterers, all of whom share responsibility for this aspect of patient care.

THERAPEUTIC DIETETICS

Therapeutic diets have an important role in modern medicine and their overall benefits have been mentioned earlier in this chapter. All persons requiring a medically prescribed, therapeutic diet, of whatever nature, need expert advice and instruction from a dietitian. In general, strict and rigid adherence to a dietary regimen, with foods having to be weighed, is seldom necessary. Many people who require dietary treatments for chronic disease may do so for a long time and often for life. Dietary restrictions may prove difficult and irksome. In view of this, any diet must be carefully adjusted to meet the needs of the individual.

UNPROVEN OR COMPLEMENTARY DIETARY THERAPIES

The practices of these dietary therapies are many and varied, and it would be impossible to discuss, in the course of this chapter, all the variations found. As one of their most common uses is in degenerative or life-threatening conditions, such as cancer or AIDS, the types of diet often recommended for these conditions are discussed below.

Most regimes share the same common principles:

- strict vegetarian or vegan diets;
- large amounts of raw foods, especially vegetables;
- sugar free;
- low fat;
- low salt;
- use of vegetable or fruit juices;
- high doses of vitamins and/or minerals.

Although some of these principles are the same as those for general healthy eating, it is the severity of these diets which sets them apart.

The macrobiotic dietary approach has the following basic principles:

- At least 50 per cent of the volume of each meal should be whole cereal grains.
- Approximately 5 per cent of daily food intake by volume should include soup (miso soup).
- About 20–30 per cent of each meal may include vegetables which should be locally grown and in season.
- 10–15 per cent of daily intake should include cooked beans and seaweed.
- Beverages should include twig tea, dandelion tea or cereal grain teas or coffees.
- A small volume of white meat or fish may be eaten once or twice a week.
- A cooked fruit dessert may be eaten two or three times a week.
- Roasted seeds, roasted nuts or dried fruit may be taken as a snack.
- Cooking oil should be of vegetable origin.
- Salt used should be unrefined sea salt.

These are only the general principles, specific diets for specific disorders will vary slightly from this.

There are other, less severe unproven dietary therapies in use which, instead of advocating an entire diet, suggest the use of certain particular foodstuffs. Examples are:

- ginseng, honey or bees' royal jelly to restore vigour and enhance well-being;
- garlic or cider vinegar to detoxify the body;
- lecithin as a slimming aid;
- linseed oil for arthritis.

It must be stressed that all persons following, or wishing to follow, any unproven dietary therapy should consult a qualified dietitian for expert advice.

Summary

The subject of nutritional therapy is a vast one. It can be seen that nutritional therapy is a vital supportive therapy in both health and disease. Although the term *nutritional therapy* may be quite new, the science is not. It is important to realise that the scope and range of the application of nutritional therapy is enormous and is not confined to the area of complementary therapies. The scientific basis and reliability of nutritional therapies varies greatly, and research is always pushing the boundaries of its usage further. However, more research is needed, especially in the area of the unproven or complementary regimes, difficult though this will be. In any case, a qualified, registered practitioner should be sought in order that sound, balanced information and advice will be provided.

References

1   R. Hutchinson and V. H. Mottram, **Food and the Principles of Dietetics**, *London: Edward Arnold*, 1933.

2   S. Davies and A. Stewart, **Nutritional Medicine**, *London: Pan*, 1987.

3   The King's Fund Working Party, **A Positive Approach to Nutrition as Treatment**, *London: King's Fund Centre*, 1992.

4   R. Passmore and M. A. Eastwood, **Human Nutrition and Dietetics**, *Edinburgh: Churchill Livingstone*, 1986.

5   WHO Study Group, **Diet, Nutrition and the Prevention of Chronic Diseases**, *Geneva: World Health Organisation*, 1990.

6   Ibid.

7   M. Hunter, Unproven dietary methods of treatment in oncology patients, In H.J. Senn, A. Glaus and L. Schmid (eds), **Supportive Care in Cancer Patients, Recent Results in Cancer Research**, (1988) 108:235.

8   Committee on Medical Aspects of Food Policy, **Dietary Reference Values for Food Energy and Nutrients for the United Kingdom**, *London: HMSO*, 1991.

9   National Advisory Committee on Nutrition Education, 'Proposals for nutritional guidelines for health education in Britain', *London: Health Education Council*, 1983.

10 Committee on Medical Aspects of Food Policy, **Diet and Cardiovascular Disease**, *London: HMSO*, 1984.

Further Reading

Any of the above reference material and the following:

H. Aihara, **Basic Macrobiotics**, *New York: Japan Publications*, 1985.

P. Fisher and A. Bender, **The Value of Food**, *Oxford: Oxford University Press*, 1975.

Health Education Authority, **Healthy Eating**, *London: HEA*, 1991.

I. Skypala, **Healthy Eating**, *London: Wisebuy*, 1988.

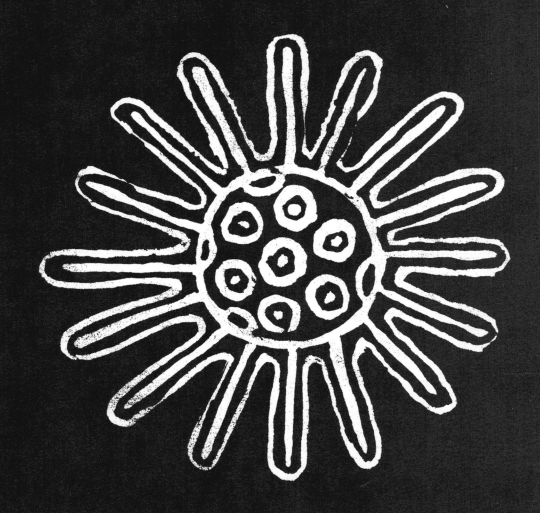

2

THE ARTS IN HEALTH CARE

Ray Rowden

Have you ever sat in the theatre or concert hall and felt your spine tingle with the breathtaking excitement of a great performance? Have you been in the cinema and wept at a powerful film? Have you enjoyed a good sing-along in a pub or a music hall? Have you tinkled around on the piano or some other instrument and enjoyed the pure fun of making music? Have you ever sat and created a rough sketch or admired a great painting for hours in a gallery, wondering what human energies and emotions lay behind the brush which adorned a canvas?

Have you boogied all night at a disco, waltzed serenely around a ballroom floor, or been through the rigours of a ballet class and experienced the sheer exhilaration of movement for movement's sake? Have you ever created something in clay or plasticine, or touched a piece of sculpture? Have you ever hit a bad time in life and released your emotions through your pen, or known a significant piece of poetry?

If you have witnessed none of these things you are probably in a minority. The arts are sometimes portrayed as being distant, somehow not relevant to daily experience in living. Nothing is further from the truth. Art, in the broadest sense, has a place in all our lives. Imagine a world without music, without colour, without literature, without song. What a barren and sterile existence we would have to endure. Art touches all our lives in thousands of different ways.

All that artistic experience has to offer is available as a potent tool in the armoury of therapy. This chapter is about harnessing and using the arts in a practical way. If you are looking for a chapter about theory, read no further – this is primarily about ideas, and information, and doing. Some of the theoretical underpinning of the rationale of the arts in health care are examined in this chapter, but it is intended to spark off your own ideas and to encourage you to try your own schemes in your own work setting.

The potential of the arts in bringing something special to those faced with sickness or chronic ill health knows no bounds. The limits are those we set. There is every reason for a sense of order and routine in the life of an institution, but there is no reason why that world cannot be touched by the richness, the beauty and the joy that the arts can offer.

A selection
of art works

In this section the reader is asked to consider what benefit the arts can provide to people in hospitals. The examples offered represent a small sample of personal experience. At the basic level the arts provide pure diversion, relief from boredom and lots of fun in a world where pleasure is sometimes lacking. The examples provided here illustrate how the arts can help people in a more profound and practical sense. These examples also cover a range of different care settings, using different art forms.

JOHN

John was a thirty-year-old who was severely mentally handicapped. In addition to this he was psychotic and experienced painful hallucinations. He spent virtually all of his life in a large mental hospital. Most of his care was provided on one ward, which had a rigid and fixed routine. The ward was run on regimented lines, with little room for people to develop their own initiative. Discipline for bad behaviour was certainly strict, and John had probably received physical punishment in his past experience.

Routine on the ward was almost suffocating. Entertainment in the ward consisted of television, radio, industrial work and an occasional trip to the hospital social centre. After a reorganisation of wards John was moved to a more enlightened environment. He had always been treated as being incapable and had a history of violent outbursts, usually linked to hallucinatory experience.

On his new ward he came into contact with imaginative nursing staff and a young occupational therapist. Over a period of a year he was gradually introduced to new experiences, such as regular trips outside the ward, usually alone or in small groups. He was also encouraged to develop his own potential in daily living activities and in caring for his personal hygiene. He responded well to a different regime. Over the months it was discovered that he loved to draw and paint. His initial work was limited, but it was evident that he took great pleasure in creating pictures. His intellect was severely limited, but through painting he found an easy way to self-expression.

His work improved, and he would spend many hours occupying himself with paints and paper. His options for activity were limited by his disability, and were compounded by years of rigid institutionalisation. Painting provided a release, and within months of taking up painting his general behaviour showed marked improvement. His confidence in himself grew and his social skills improved.

During his hallucinatory episodes, when he became violent, he had to be segregated from others, for his own safety and that of other people. After an episode of aggression he would remain sultry for many hours.

Painting afforded a solution to this problem. After he had begun to paint he was encouraged to pick up his brushes as soon as he could after an hallucinatory experience where violence had occurred. This led to a much quicker return to his usual happy disposition.

The general milieu of his new ward undoubtedly contributed much to the improvement in John's quality of life, but the introduction of painting to his range of experience was a vital and useful part of his total care.

MARTIN

Martin was a sixteen-year-old who was in hospital for radiotherapy for a brain tumour. Prior to the diagnosis of a tumour Martin had been a large, robust and happy-go-lucky individual. He adored football, and regularly attended matches. His tumour presented with an epileptiform seizure, which was investigated. He was immediately admitted to hospital and underwent extensive surgery to remove the tumour. He went into the operating theatre an active sixteen-year-old. He came out minus his brain tumour but with some severe neurological problems, including a left-sided hemiparesis.

After recovery from surgery he was transferred to a second hospital for five weeks of radiotherapy. His home life was far from stable. His mother had remarried following divorce and the relationship between Martin and his stepfather was stormy. After the diagnosis of his tumour Martin's mother became very anxious and over-protective, giving up her job to devote all her time to her son. Martin's stepfather resented this.

In the second hospital Martin began radiotherapy and an active programme of physiotherapy and occupational therapy, designed to return mobility and to improve his co-ordination and finer hand movement. He became a problem. Over the first week of his stay he began to miss radiotherapy treatments, and he would not attend the physiotherapy or occupational therapy departments regularly. He frequently absented himself from the hospital without permission, and at this stage his gait was far from secure.

In the ward he became abusive and threatening towards other patients and towards nursing staff. Things were rapidly moving from bad to worse, with his stepfather refusing to allow him home for weekend leaves because of his behaviour. A consultant psychiatrist was called in to see him to see if there was any underlying psychological problem requiring clinical treatment. There was not.

After the visit by the psychiatrist a case conference was called with the nurses and the occupational therapist to discuss Martin. It became obvious that Martin was perfectly normal. His behaviour was his way of kicking against a hospital regime which was denying him access to normality. Because of his mobility problems all staff were reluctant to let him out of the hospital.

He wanted to go to his youth club in the evenings, he wanted to keep contact with his football chums, and generally feared becoming an outcast from his friends and peers. All the hospital had ever said to Martin was that he was expected to comply with his treatment, which was life-saving. They repeatedly said 'no' to anything that he wanted. His reaction was to assert his presence through aggressive behaviour as he could see no other solution.

It was agreed that Martin be approached with a view to drawing up a contract between him and the ward nursing staff, and the occupational therapy department. Within the contract he was expected to deliver certain things; namely to turn up to his various therapy sessions and to behave in a reasonable fashion on the ward. In return, he was provided with a programme of activity which allowed him to go to his youth club one evening a week, and to have an occasional trip into town when staffing allowed for an escort. In addition, we negotiated with his parents to allow him home at weekends. We also attempted to find some responsible volunteers who would take him to football matches. A member of the team supporters' club agreed to do this with the proviso that Martin stayed off the terraces, which were not exactly noted for behaviour of a genteel nature!

To alleviate boredom we also agreed to provide him with a video machine in his single room and a personal stereo. He loved music and was able to bring in his own tapes from home. The hospital also had a selection of rock and pop on video, which was made available to him.

He was encouraged to come to events organised in the hospital, including concert evenings. We also negotiated for him to work in the packing room of the hospital central sterile supplies department four mornings a week.

His behaviour began to improve immediately. Within one week Martin ceased to be a problem. He was responsible for himself, and he knew it. He also knew that, despite the fact that he had to be hospitalised for long periods, it was possible to hang on to normality, although during his initial stay he did break the contract on one or two occasions.

On the first occasion he had an altercation with a nurse, using foul language, and had refused to go to the radiotherapy department for treatment. The staff were full of trepidation, but Martin was quietly advised that he had reneged on his side of the bargain and he lost his video supply for two days and missed a visit to the youth club. We all feared that he would not be able to handle this, but he did.

We also broke the bargain. Because of emergencies in the ward or last-minute sickness, sometimes what he expected could not be delivered. He was quick to remind us of our commitments and negotiated repatriation arrangements, which were always honoured. Over the following year he was to have many more admissions to the hospital, but he knew that they need not be bad experiences. He became a friend to many people in the hospital, and his treatment was successful. He is now free of disease and living happily and independently in the community. He sailed perilously close to admission to a psychiatric hospital, but a creative programme provided real solutions.

SUSAN

Susan was sixty years of age and was in hospital with widely metastasised breast disease, with neurological impairment. She was very limited in mobility and was in pain. Her mood was low and lethargic and she knew that her life expectancy was limited. She had been in hospital for some weeks and was cared for in a single room.

Her husband was loving and supportive but the ward nursing staff knew that he had experienced great strain in helping her morale. This admission had occurred around Christmas time. The main objective of care was to provide Susan with relief from pain and to encourage her to mobilise and to improve her morale.

Susan heard that two dancers from The Royal Ballet were coming to the hospital to perform just before Christmas, and showed immediate interest. The nurses recognised this and began to discuss with her the idea of getting up out of bed and attending the performance. Despite some reluctance, she was keen to try. The performance was some two weeks ahead and, working with her husband, the nurses and the physiotherapist, Susan set her sights on making it to the performance.

In discussions it was discovered that she had a great love of ballet, and had actually trained to a fairly high level of competence in her youth with a famous teacher. She was provided with a video player in her room and a variety of full-length ballets on tape. The tapes provided her with a great deal of joy, and she and her husband spent many happy hours glued to the screen.

The evening of the performance arrived and Susan was now spending

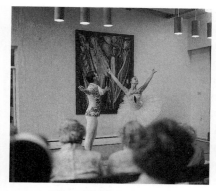
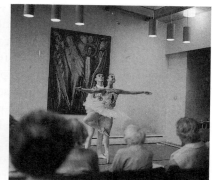
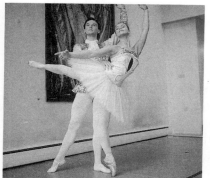
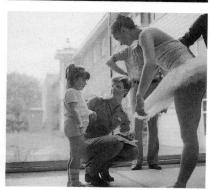

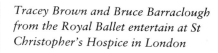
Tracey Brown and Bruce Barraclough from the Royal Ballet entertain at St Christopher's Hospice in London

much less time in her bed and was really motivated. Since this was an occasion, she arranged to have her hair set and she put on some make-up for the evening. During the show she sat at the front, transfixed, completely forgetting any discomfort.

At the conclusion of the performance she presented flowers to the dancers and was radiant. Drinks and supper were organised and the dancers remained for over an hour, chatting away with Susan about her past training and ballet in general.

For Susan, this event provided a magical experience at a crucial time. After the performance she remained motivated and free of pain. Susan died shortly after this experience. Her husband told the staff how much the event had meant to him and to Susan, and how it had made the burden of the final period of her life so much easier to bear.

TIM

Tim was twenty-three years old and had developed a testicular teratoma. He had entered hospital for initial investigations and was due to commence treatment without delay. He was admitted to a mixed medical ward where most of the patients were a good deal older than he. His anxiety levels were giving staff cause for concern. His face was taut with worry of what the future held for him, and despite information and reassurance from staff he remained painfully frightened.

During his stay a record request session was held in the music room of the hospital, where ten or twelve patients met and shared their musical tastes. The nurse caring for Tim suggested that he might like to attend. Despite initial reluctance, he went along.

In the music room was another young man who also had testicular cancer but who was on a ward where patients were more mobile and able to care for themselves. As Tim entered the music room it was obvious, from the look on his face, that he registered the presence of another patient nearer his own age. Tim made a bee line for him and began an embarrassed conversation.

Fortunately this other patient was well through treatment, understood his illness and had a positive outlook on life. Within minutes, the two of them were heavily engaged in discussion, with Tim visibly relaxing.

Through the music Tim heard other people talking about their lives and experiences, and about living with illness. During tea he and the other young patient continued to talk. This patient explained to Tim what the treatment involved and also told Tim that his own cancer was cured. To Tim the diagnosis of cancer had felt like a death sentence. He had heard various staff tell him that he had a good chance of successful treatment, but he had not really believed what he was being told. He now knew that this was the truth because he was able to hear it from someone in the same position as himself.

Tim returned to the ward in a totally different frame of mind. That evening he and his fellow patient arranged to meet, and became firm friends. Tim adjusted perfectly to his treatment and, three years later, is completely free of disease. A simple music session with records and a chance meeting made all the difference to his treatment.

Short-term care

The breast unit at the Royal Marsden Hospital in Surrey has six beds which are used for the staging of breast cancer. Each week six women who are newly diagnosed come into the hospital to assess the state of their disease, and decisions are taken about treatment.

The women in this unit are in for a stay of only three or four days. They undergo a barrage of tests and investigations and are seen by a host of doctors, technicians, nurse specialists and others. The hospital has a regular programme of live music, provided by the Council for Music in Hospitals, and a variety of other live performances.

When this programme was started it was thought that the longer-term patients would derive benefit from the programme, but it was found that newly admitted women from the breast unit were attending. On investigation it was found that the evening housekeeper on the ward always made sure that the newly admitted women knew what shows were on, and she would encourage them to attend and escort them up to the area where performances were given.

On talking to numerous women at concerts it became obvious how valuable this was. A number of these women came into hospital, having had previous admissions elsewhere, and were quite surprised to find that a concert was provided, together with facilities for socialising afterwards.

On countless occasions they commented on how this activity relaxed them totally and removed the fear of hospital. The evening also allowed them to meet each other socially and facilitated a sense of friendship between them, which has proved valuable on many occasions.

Short-term or acute care patients can enjoy this type of activity as much as people who are in for a longer stay.

CAPTAIN H

Captain H was 72 years old and was in hospital for treatment of a major illness, but he also suffered from an arthritic condition that gave him great pain. He was an ex-Army man, tall and proud, and found the whole business of illness difficult to bear, but was determined to keep a stiff upper lip.

His illness had reduced his mobility, and hospitalisation, coupled with his treatments, did not make movement any easier. His arthritic condition deteriorated and his pain was becoming more of a problem. He confided to his nurse that his pain was not controlled, and steps were taken to alter his drugs. Over the following week a variety of alterations were made, all to no avail.

Stronger analgesics were tried, but Captain H did not like the notion of stronger drugs and disliked the side effects. After this, it was decided that acupuncture might be of value and a course of treatment began, again to no avail. His wife reported to his nurse that she was worried as the pain was becoming worse, even with greater mobilisation, and that he was getting very depressed but not showing this.

The nurse discussed this with Captain H and asked the occupational therapist to see him. The occupational therapist was skilled in relaxation techniques and used a variety of tapes. Captain H was extremely sceptical about the notion of relaxation. The occupational therapist discovered that he liked music and explored his tastes, which were distinctly classical. Using a mixture of her tapes and his, she devised a plan for relaxation.

Captain H and she would use a quiet room, with the blinds drawn, and she gradually withdrew until he had mastered the technique himself. In no time at all his pain was controlled. He actually cut down his analgesia and would use relaxation techniques whenever he experienced pain. He refined the technique to the point where he could gain total relaxation to his favourite music.

MICHELLE

Michelle was thirteen when she was removed from her home to an adolescent unit in a psychiatric hospital. Her home background was difficult, with divorced parents and a mother who brought into her life many different boyfriends. In Michelle's life violence was almost an everyday event.

It was discovered that Michelle had been skipping school nearly every day for more than a year. She would attend in the morning and register, then slip away. She had also forged various notes in her mother's name, providing her with an explanation for various absences from school. When not at school she became involved in petty theft, vandalism and solvent abuse.

Michelle had become aggressive, fairly hard bitten and was phobic about school. In an attempt to place a protective wall around her fragile ego she built a persona based on bravado and aggression. The unit had a school attached to it, which worked with children with educational problems on an individual basis. The school had a policy that allowed the children to set their own pace in returning to school work.

In most cases youngsters would gradually build themselves up to a return to normal patterns of education, and would begin this process within a matter of days. In Michelle's case it was to take much longer. Despite careful groundwork with Michelle involving nurses, doctors and teachers, she would make no attempt to attend the school attached to the unit.

Her behaviour was belligerent and she showed all the signs of being an arch-manipulator of weaker personalities, and she became a natural leader in any group. Her leadership did not encourage socially acceptable behaviour and she was frequently found bullying or hitting weaker children.

After five weeks Michelle had made no attempt to step inside the school. Her days were spent aimlessly, often in front of the television, but more often than not she would simply mope around.

One day some of the other children returned to the unit from the school clutching some mugs they had made in the pottery studio. Possession of a mug was perceived as something of a status symbol, with much banter as to who had created the best product. Michelle stayed on the fringes but was definitely interested in knowing more about the pottery studio.

One of the teachers invited her over to the school to look at the facilities. The school boasted a well-equipped studio with a wide variety of wheels and kilns, as well as facilities for sculpture of various kinds.

Michelle, attempting to maintain her defences, put on an air of total lack of interest but reluctantly agreed to give pottery a try. The following day she spent the morning at the potter's wheel. The teacher worked with her and found that she had a natural flair for working with clay. As the days passed Michelle created some outstanding work at the potter's wheel. Her work drew instant attention since her eye for colour and design was instinctive.

Her confidence began to build and she was soon absorbing books on pottery and sculpture. After her initial encounter with the wheel she branched out into creating figurines in clay and also worked with other materials. She soon had an impressive collection, some of which were exhibited in a local show.

Through creative work she gradually began a slow reintroduction to general education, building one step at a time. Michelle eventually left the unit and returned to normality outside hospital and a school with a pottery studio, where a sound arts curriculum was found that was willing to accept her.

Why art?

Illness isolates people. Consider what health-care systems do to the individual, particularly in an institutional setting of any kind. The business of becoming ill, on any level, is traumatic and the process of 'becoming a patient' is, all too often, destined to strip away our individuality.

If we take an acute care setting we find a busy environment that is cure-orientated, into which humans are taken at a vulnerable time in life. The individual is then gradually saturated into a foreign sub-culture where the language of the professional rules. In many subtle ways we begin to push the individual into a passive role. In recent years there has been a move towards the provision of individualised care, but how often is individual care sacrificed on the altar of institutional convenience?

We take individuals, and usually the first thing we do in a ward or clinic is to deprive them of their clothes. We then proceed to elicit personal details about their life, recording a multitude of data on a file which is, in most settings, kept in the hands of the professional. After this they will probably be subjected to a barrage of tests and investigations, and ultimately treated.

As if illness, its effects and the whole business of treatment were not enough to cope with, we also pin the individuals to our routines. Whatever the individual lifestyle of the patients, to some extent they will be automatically expected to gear themselves to our routines. In many instances this is unavoidable because of external pressure on hospital personnel, but do we always recognise what the business of 'becoming a patient' actually means to the individual?

Let us examine what life in the average acute hospital is like. In most settings we will expect our patients to share a bedroom, in some cases with up to twenty or more other people. The environment and routine will be geared totally towards illness, diagnosis and treatment. On a basic level the day will be broken by activities related to what the professionals dictate, punctuated mainly by meal times and beverages, again set by the institution.

In some settings we will rigidly dictate when our patients can be visited by their loved ones and by other significant people in their lives. Worse still, we may even find wards that will attempt to order life even more rigidly, telling our patients when they must lie down, when they must get up, and in some instances when they can use a bedpan or take a bath. In essence, we take people out of their normality and impose upon them abnormality, and we do it at the very time they need their normality most.

If we consider long-stay care settings, the picture can be equally bleak. In the United Kingdom many thousands of people who are elderly, mentally ill or handicapped, or physically disabled are cared for in institutions large and small. In many settings life for people in care can be dull and unimaginative. When we examine the reasons for this it has to be recognised that under-funding plays a significant part in the style and the flavour of care provided.

In a ward with thirty aged women, half of whom are doubly incontinent, all demented, how can we expect three or four nurses to provide creative care regimes that take into account the individual? All too often the relentless boredom of long-stay care is dictated by a lack of resources, financial and human.

In a setting where staff are stretched to the limit, coping behaviour is easily adopted. It is easier, for example, for one nurse to feed six patients rather than allow time for all patients to try to feed themselves. It becomes logistically easier to put fifteen patients through the bathroom on a conveyor-belt system. It is less hassle to put milk, sugar and tea into a communal teapot, rather than allow time to let the individual find his or her limits and capabilities. The pressures inherent in an institution which is under-resourced are all destined to deny the individuals choices in life, both at a basic and on a much deeper level.

Being a patient, in any setting, can be a thoroughly boring experience. Too often we are guilty of sensory deprivation on an almost scandalous scale. We isolate people from society, from their own norms, and provide a living environment that is desperately abnormal, where sensitivities become blunted and blurred, and we do this in the name of health care. Basic boredom is a problem that the arts, in all forms, can tackle in an imaginative and exciting way.

On a deeper level, institutional care, particularly in situations where a long stay in hospital is involved, can damage the individual in a profound sense. Ask yourself what you would do if you were plucked from your normal lifestyle and placed in the care of an institution for three months. Imagine what it means to someone who may be cut off for years.

Institutionalisation and its effects are well documented; we know that it can lead to all kinds of 'abnormal' behaviour – is it any wonder? What we witness in the person who becomes institutionalised is the eventual outcome of the process of loss of individuality, of knowing 'what is me'.

A creative regime that uses the arts can restore to a person a sense of individuality and reality. In the drab and lonely world of the person in institutional care art can speak of beauty, of emotion, of feeling, of human richness, for the way in which each of us responds to creative stimuli is totally unique. The arts can act as a powerful catalyst which allows each of us to identify something in ourselves that is ours and ours alone, but that can be shared and enjoyed with others, as we choose.

In many cases, health-care professionals only see a place for the arts and other types of diversional activity in long-stay care, particularly with the aged, the mentally ill and the handicapped. This view misses one vital aspect of the value of arts. In many settings, including acute care, the arts have a potential to assist the process of healing.

There is a large volume of research into the healing value of the arts, particularly music, but consider also the clinical evidence that is available to support the use of creative activity and its link to healing. *Healing* is a term that has wide meaning, and the arts can heal in every sense – spiritual, emotional and physical.

The study of psychosomatic medicine provides us with ample evidence of the importance of the link between mind and body. The human mind is complex, and despite the obvious wisdom of Western medicine, there remains much that we do not begin to understand. But consider what we do know: there are a variety of physical illnesses which are caused in part by psychological factors or, when present, are maintained by psychological factors. Examples of these conditions are many cases of gastro-intestinal ulcers, bronchial asthma, colitis and a variety of skin conditions.

Modern theory suggests that people who suffer from psychosomatic conditions have problems in maintaining their own internal emotional equilibrium, which leads to physiological manifestations of ill health.

Another example of the vital link between mind and body is provided in the examination of hysterical neurosis involving conversion. In people who experience this condition the mind is quite capable of producing physical symptoms of a wide variety, where the individual's mental turmoil finds a physical means of expression. Conversion hysteria can produce blindness, deafness, paralysis of various types, spasm of ocular muscles, fits, tics, tumours, mutism and a whole range of other conditions. The psyche is powerful in its influence on health and is quite capable of influencing physiological balance.

At a more basic level we know that the person confronted with illness who is positive, alert and in a healthy frame of mind is more likely to recover quickly. In the care of people with cancer, the link between good mental health and recovery and coping with treatment is well recognised and is receiving greater attention in research centres around the world.

In situations where people have physical disability, and where mobility is important, the patient's emotional state is crucial to the development of a successful rehabilitation plan. If the elderly person in care is institutionalised and lethargic, there is little chance of returning to a normal independent lifestyle. There is no doubt that our mental health influences our reactions to physical ill health. The arts can be very powerful in helping the individual towards recovery from illness and can be used as a wholly practical tool in the rehabilitation armoury in *any* setting where care is provided.

A well-thought-through arts programme can offer a healthy means of escape from clinical dominance of life. In many instances, ill health leads to individuals thinking that they are alone in their experience. Aside from social intercourse in a ward, patients and their families have little opportunity to meet normally. A forced chat at visiting times may be all that some hospitalised people experience. In some instances, patients in a ward will share experiences, exchange anecdotes and often do more harm than good.

Activity within an arts programme can, and does, facilitate a sharing of experience for patients and families in a healthy and productive way. The provision of activity related to non-clinical, non-disease spheres of life can act as an oasis of natural and free communication between patients and families that can do much to dispel isolation and loneliness.

A concert evening, watching slides, videos and so on, followed by something to eat and drink, can allow patients to come together as people. Such activity can free patients from all the trappings that go to make up the experience of 'being a patient'. Staff can also be on hand (preferably out of uniform) and share in the normality of patients and their families, and guide where misconception occurs.

Do we really ever allow enough time for this type of communication to take place in our busy professional world? It is unrealistic to imagine that the average general hospital would be able to provide group therapy on a regular basis. It is also, to some extent, natural that hospitals by definition will place the greatest emphasis on investigation, treatment and cure. Arts activities can be an easy and natural way of improving the environment in which patients are cared for, and can do so much to say to each individual, 'You may be ill, you may be in hospital, but above all *be yourself.*'

Art is therapeutic in the widest and truest sense, and is as natural to people as the air we breathe. Art is not highbrow or for an elite; it has the power to speak to all. If we look back in history we find countless examples of people wanting to express themselves creatively, from the cave dwellers who had the inspiration to paint murals reflecting their day-to-day life, to prisoners in Nazi concentration camps who used music, writing, painting and other art forms to cling onto a small spark of humanity in the carnage of the Holocaust.

Art is fundamental to the nature of being. Each of us has the ability to create, however simply we choose to do it. We can all sing a note, draw a picture, shape a piece of clay, or respond to a great performance in a way that no one else can. The need for people to be creative in our world, dominated as it is by technology and instant entertainment, is easily overlooked.

Yet it is at times of adversity, as in illness, when we are cut off from reality, that creative activity can offer most. Health-care workers are in a natural position to open doors for people in their care, and a door to creative experience can be as therapeutic and as valuable as any drug, operation or curative intervention.

Resources in health care are always limited, but imagination knows no limits and a little can go a long way towards making the experience of the individual in hospital less traumatic and in providing care which is genuinely holistic.

What can you do?

Many health-care professionals – nurses, doctors, occupational therapists and others – may live and work in areas that are some distance from a major centre of population. This need not preclude the establishment of a modest but vibrant programme of arts. One thing that we can thank technology for is the rapid development of high-quality entertainment equipment at reasonable prices, which can make the arts easily accessible. Perhaps the reader can absorb some ideas that can be applied in any care setting in any part of the country from this chapter. All that is really needed is an electricity supply, goodwill and enthusiasm.

Canned music

In modern life we are often assaulted by a barrage of sound, much of it meaningless. If we go to the airport terminal, to a hotel lobby, or to buy a tin of peas from the supermarket, we frequently find background music designed to lull the listener. In hospitals we can often find an even more bizarre mix of sounds. Have you ever walked into a hospital ward and found the most inappropriate music being forced into everyone's ears; for example, Radio 1 blaring out of a ward radio, delivering a constant supply of pop music to elderly people?

Music needs careful thought. Use of the radio can be valuable in a controlled way. A scan of the weekly programmes is often worthwhile as it may reveal forthcoming broadcasts which can be discussed with patients with a view to planned listening, which is particularly useful in long-stay settings, and provides an opportunity to reinforce individual choice for patients. A radio relentlessly blaring out sound in an open ward rarely has any value, and can do harm. How can a constant barrage of sound be of value to a confused elderly person?

The choice of radio programmes, or for that matter TV viewing, is often automatically made by staff, imposing staff tastes onto patients. The radio offers access to a wide range of musical tastes. Discussion with patients, coupled with sensible planning, can cater for all. There may even be occasions when elderly people might want to listen to pop music, but they should have the choice. Periods of silence are also needed!

Music
systems

A high-quality stereo system has great application in a ward or clinic. One dentist has a stereo installed in his practice and he allows patients to bring in their own records, which is a marvellous asset to patients who are anxious. In hospitals, a music system can provide a life-line.

Not only can a ward or department build its own library, but people can also be actively encouraged to bring in music of their own choice. For people who regularly have to come to an outpatient's clinic, having their own choice of music can make the experience much easier to bear.

People who need regular dialysis or chemotherapy or who need to be attached to a cell separator will often have time on their hands. A portable stereo or fixed system can provide a lot of pleasure. The ward sound system should also be provided with headphones, which will allow people to listen in private, without any disturbance to others.

Records and tapes can be used imaginatively. Music is important to most people. We all tend to link particular pieces of music to an important event in our lives or to an important period of life. This can be easily arranged. A nurse, occupational therapist, or even a good volunteer, can go round to patients and ask if they have a piece of music they would particularly like to hear. If the hospital has a radio station, records and tapes containing the patients' choices can be obtained.

If there is no hospital radio station, most libraries now have an extensive selection of records and tapes, and your local librarian may be more than willing to provide a special service for hospital patients. Having identified requests, groups of patients can be brought together to share their choices in an afternoon or evening session, rounded off with tea or other refreshments.

It is amazing what this kind of activity can offer. People will often want to talk about their choice of music and will discuss its significance with a small group of people, which can reveal facets of personality that have been totally unseen. Record request sessions can also be an easy way of making the day more varied.

Walkmans

Mini stereo cassette-players offer a revolution to patients who are immobile or bedridden. Hospital radio ear sets are notorious for their poor quality. When one is ill it is imperative that quality in sound is provided, and personal stereo provides an ideal solution. Two or three of these in a ward will usually be sufficient, and patients can be encouraged to bring in their own.

Personal stereo allows the patients to enjoy their own choice of music that is high in quality and to cause no disturbance to others. Wards or hospitals can build their own libraries, and patients and visitors can be encouraged to bring tapes from home. People of all age ranges can benefit from such a service, but it is particularly valuable to patients who are in isolation for any length of time and to those who are confined to bed or chair.

Security can be a problem, so the marking of equipment and a record of loans should be thought through before introducing such a service. It is also important to have an adequate supply of changeable ear pads so that fresh sets can be put on the headphones for each person. A short soak in disinfectant between use will usually be sufficient to prevent cross-infection. In patients with serious infection ear pads have to be destroyed, but fortunately they are inexpensive.

Video

Video players are often plentiful in hospitals, usually in the education centre. A video machine can prove of immense value in any ward.

Patients can be encouraged to bring in their own material, or relatives can hire tapes. A day room is the best place for a video player, where it can be used at any time, day or night, without causing a nuisance to anyone. Again, many local libraries will stock pre-recorded videos and provide a special service to the local hospital.

Alternatively, video rental shops may be prepared to allow your ward or department specially reduced rates or even supply you without charge. Video playback facilities can also have a value in outpatient's clinics; for example, where children are congregated a programme can be geared to their needs. This is much better than waiting with nothing to do. Videos in clinic areas can also be used to transmit health education material.

A machine mounted on a portable trolley can also have a place. If a patient with a minority interest wishes to watch a programme, a trolley-mounted machine, preferably with headphones, can be taken easily to the bedside. There is an excellent stock of opera, ballet and music on video which can be obtained easily, thus catering for all tastes.

Pop videos can also be appreciated by younger patients on a trolley-mounted machine. Patients in strict isolation can find a private video machine a godsend. Remember to allow for the sexual needs of strictly isolated patients. If you are isolated for a long period sexual gratification is pretty limited. Isolated patients, both men and women, have been known to request some fairly risqué material, and a private video provides a reasonable solution. You may not consider the blue movie an art form, but there are some who hold a contrary view!

Video equipment can provide an alternative television channel. Your engineering staff may be able to link a video player into the main TV aerial system of the hospital, linking the machine to every TV set in the wards. Through such a system a whole alternative viewing programme can be established. Programming can be geared to meet the needs of particular groups of people. At the Royal Marsden Hospital this system has been in operation for some years. The programme provides something for everyone.

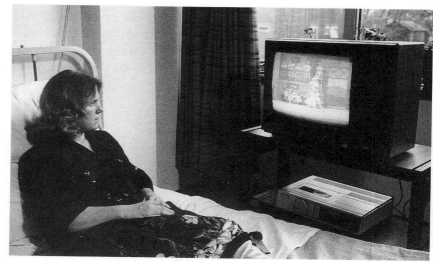

Personal video can offer access to a wide range of arts from the bedside

EXAMPLE OF SCHEDULE

Monday to Friday – 0700–0900 hours: children's material
Monday to Friday – 1400 hours: matinée movie
Monday to Friday – 2300 hours: late night movie
At the weekends and on bank holidays a selection of programmes
will be screened.

A centrally placed video allows you total flexibility in programme setting and the hospital electrician or engineering staff may prove willing volunteers in making the scheme work. A centrally placed machine can also allow for a request system to operate. At the Royal Marsden Hospital all wards have a supply of request forms for patients.

The form is completed, stating what video is wanted and the screening time requested. This is sent to the engineers' department. The staff then order the request from the video supplier. The video machine can then be pre-set to deliver individual requests at the time which suits the patient.

Video can also be used to create a special occasion. At holiday times special showings can be arranged when the hospital can be very quiet. A day room can be set aside and an opera or ballet can then be shown. This may be particularly popular at Christmas and on bank holiday weekends.

In one place these occasions were organised for the evenings and patients were always encouraged to dress and to bring along visitors. The room was filled with flowers, the walls decorated with posters. An interval was always planned, where wine and a buffet was served. On special occasions champagne would be provided. In addition to opera or ballet, great cinema classics can make an occasion special, and give a patient in hospital a real sense of contact with the world beyond the hospital.

Guest speakers

A speaker invited into the hospital can provide a breath of fresh air to hospital life, and it is amazing what talent exists in your local community if you go out and look. Any professional artist who is articulate can provide a fascinating half hour, sharing life's experiences with patients. Equally, people skilled in crafts or handiwork can be absorbing, particularly if audience involvement and participation is encouraged.

Specialist speakers, such as police officers involved in interesting work, or other service providers who can give a look behind the scenes of their world, are popular. This can really take a person out of the world of hospitals in a practical sense. Local community groups such as Rotary Clubs, Lions Clubs and Women's Institutes can provide a valuable source of speakers.

On the whole, people are more than willing to provide this service without charge. Great care needs to be taken in the use of speakers. Remember, your audience is captive and deserves excellence. A speaker who is not properly vetted or prepared might prove to be a disaster. A weekly or fortnightly guest provides a valuable addition to any arts programme.

Crafts

Traditional craft work in occupational therapy has been around for a long time and has become the subject of many jokes. We all know of the popular myth of the occupational therapist as the 'basket weaving lady', whose sole task is the provision of craft work. To an extent hospitals have in the past relied too heavily on this type of activity. It has, however, great value and allows people to create something, born of their own skill and ability.

A good stock of equipment for simple craft work is useful in any ward or department. A sewing box, knitting equipment, crocheting, macramé, basket weaving and other simple activities can offer people a creative activity. In long-stay settings much more sophistication is called for, and the variety of craft works offered should be as wide as possible.

Sports

Sports activities in hospital settings of all kinds are valuable. Most hospitals have an area where a ball can be kicked around, as a release for energy, for good exercise and basic relief from the boredom of routine. A basic selection of sports equipment can be a real asset. Indoor equipment is also useful, and an area in the hospital that has a table tennis set and a small pool or billiards table will rarely be out of use. This will also provide a centre where natural communication between people can occur.

Gardening

Making things grow, particularly at a time of worry, discomfort or adversity, is deeply creative, and much pleasure is derived from watching things grow. An area of the hospital grounds set aside for patients is worth considering, where people can potter around or do some serious gardening. On the ward, particularly in inner-city areas, window boxes, tubs and an attractive selection of house plants can enhance the atmosphere of any clinical setting and allow patients to become involved in creating growth. Grow-bags also offer a flexible alternative where space is a problem.

Music rooms

In most hospitals space is at a premium, but a room set aside for music is a good investment. Obviously, in ideal settings a music room should be sound-proofed. Where this is not possible try to find a room that is not too close to areas where very ill patients are cared for. With a music room your imagination can run wild, but a basic stock of instruments can be readily available.

A music room should contain popular instruments such as piano and guitar, and access should be available to simple woodwind instruments. Instruments can be fixed to the wall by the use of reinforced steel wire, which is light and flexible. In addition to a range of instruments, a high-quality stereo sound system with headphones can find a natural home in a music room.

Many people enjoy making music and, if you are talented as a musician, coming into a hospital with the facilities to use your skill can offer a great deal of pleasure. If a patient is a skilled musician he or she may even generate interest by providing entertainment for other patients, visitors and staff. In addition to instruments provided, patients can be encouraged to bring in their own, although that may present problems to the harpist or bass player! Instruments are expensive, but funds spent in this area can offer great rewards.

Live performance

There is nothing quite like the magic that can be woven by live performance. Where it is not possible to use the skills of professionals, for reasons of finance or geography, it is worthwhile seeking out talented amateurs in your own locality.

The range of performance is vast in all the visual and performing arts, including music, dance, song, drama, poetry recitals, mime and many others. A word of caution: never use an artist whom you have not auditioned. Talented amateurs can be exceptionally skilled, but they can also be embarrassing.

Communicating the joy of art with people is a highly skilled activity, communicating with the sick or disabled even more so. Amateur performance can have a value, but proceed with care and thought. Local music groups, drama groups and arts associations are often willing to participate in work in hospitals, and can provide a source of talented artists. Children are nearly always welcome visitors to the world of the hospital.

Local groups such as the Guides or Scouts may be happy to come into the hospital and put on a simple show. Likewise, local youth clubs, upper schools and dance schools can offer you a wide choice of live performances. Great care needs to be taken in liaison with amateur groups, particularly with children, and preparation of the performers is essential since they may not know what to expect in a hospital.

Ward-based
activity

Think about equipment that is around your own ward or department. How often have you sat in a waiting room and read tatty magazines, all of the same type and usually way out of date. A little thought can transform your ward or department. Reading material in common living areas is important to people with time on their hands. A wide selection of magazines, covering different subjects, will get a great deal of use. Staff members can be asked to bring in fresh supplies, and it can often be a useful learning experience for a student nurse to take responsibility for this aspect of provision.

A small library of books can also be of real benefit on the ward, particularly where there is no hospital library. Even when a library service is available, it will usually be open at set times and not in the evenings, at weekends and over holiday periods. An imaginative small selection of books on the ward is appreciated.

Your local book shops or secondhand shops may prove more than willing to help you with supplies, and staff may be prepared to bring in books that they no longer wish to keep. In so many wards and departments a sparse selection of reading material is left around with little or no thought. Being hospitalised and faced with a tatty selection of nothing but back numbers of *Punch* or nothing but westerns or detective stories to read is not exactly conducive to the creative use of spare time. Health education material can be kept with or near more general reading material, and is likely to get far more use in this setting.

Board games, packs of cards and jigsaws may not fall purely under the heading of arts, but do think about the stock carried on your ward or what is available around the hospital. Games and jigsaws can provide endless hours of pleasure. A well-kept stock is always a valuable asset to life on the ward.

In long-stay settings photography has great value in the life of a ward. If your patients go on outings or have celebrations, a picture gallery that captures their lives is much appreciated. You may not have a Lord Lichfield or a David Bailey on your ward but photographic art is easy, and a staff member or an able patient who is skilled with a camera can enrich life and create a colourful display.

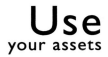

Use
your assets

In the average ward there are a variety of staff, including nurses, paramedical staff, doctors, porters, housekeeping staff, members of the League of Friends and students of all kinds passing through. All of these staff have a life outside their work and could be harbouring the most amazing gifts.

Find out about staff hobbies, any trips abroad or at home that are planned, or any major life events such as a wedding or a new baby, that might be shared with patients. Simple and popular hobbies, such as stamp collecting, amateur photography or musical skills lend themselves readily to sharing with patients, both in large and small groups, and on a one-to-one basis.

Staff time can also be used creatively. In many hospitals of all kinds, nursing and other care staff can almost feel guilty if they are not seen to be 'busy'. How many nurses remember cleaning the sluice for the fifth time because the nursing officer was on the ward and things were quiet! This really is a criminal waste of time. In all settings nurses and others should use time to communicate.

Activities which harness the power of the arts can allow natural communication to occur between patients and staff. One young staff nurse was seen playing a game of Scrabble with three patients: an elderly lady who had had her left breast removed, a young man with testicular teratoma and an anxious middle-aged man who was receiving radiotherapy for cancer of the bronchus. The conversation created by the nurse was beautiful.

Through a simple board game she was able to bring together three unlikely partners who, as the game progressed, shared their worries and fears with one another and with their nurse. Nothing was forced; it all happened perfectly naturally. The patients were in the care of a nurse who used her time creatively – much more beneficial than cleaning the cupboards or the sluice for the nth time.

We need to remember that holistic care calls for more than the mere acquisition of clinical skills and involves more than the giving of clinical treatments. Care staff who are sensitive to the total needs of people and who are not inhibited by outdated thinking can bring the value of communication to their day-to-day work in simple but effective ways that need not detract from the routine needs of the institution.

Preparation

Regardless of the activity concerned, investment in preparation is an essential ingredient to a successful programme of any kind. Staff in hospitals need a full understanding of what arts activities are capable of achieving and what is involved. If staff remain aloof, uninterested or impose their own negative views, this is transmitted to patients.

It is essential that a programme is broadly based, reflecting a variety of tastes. It is never excusable to impose your own bias onto a captive audience. A catholic taste is an asset, as is the ability to sit through activities that you might personally detest, yet attempt to share the enjoyment of others.

The involvement of staff in all activities is vital, allowing them to share experience with patients on a human level. It is not always possible for this to occur, particularly in busy acute settings. Intelligent and informed staff can, however, provide patients with positive encouragement, even if they are too busy actually to join in.

Preparation of the environment in which programmes take place also requires planning. If you are providing your patients with a guest speaker or a live performance, this is best planned around the routine of the hospital. Afternoons when treatment sessions or theatre lists are less busy are more suitable for these activities. Ward staff may also need to be a little more sensitive to the noise created in the general life of the ward if a guest is sharing skills with patients.

Arts activities can teach much to students of health care from all disciplines and should be used to broaden and to enrich the learning opportunities provided. Students also have youth and enthusiasm on their side. Properly harnessed, these gifts can offer much to the success of a programme.

In an arts-orientated programme quality is always more important than quantity in terms of audience size. Nothing is more painful than witnessing patients being forced or jollied along into involvement in activities. If a programme offers quality, it will succeed. Whether it succeeds with an audience of two, or of forty-two, does not really matter. It is vital that people are not forced into participation.

Coercion totally negates the value of arts-related activity in reinforcing individuality. Many people, particularly in the United Kingdom, may be conditioned to expecting a rigid routine in hospitals, and may find it actually a culture shock to find live performance or music. Sensible discussion of a programme and gentle encouragement should be all that is needed.

In the past, hordes of long-stay psychiatric patients would be marshalled to various activities in a vast hall. If someone is forced into activities with no real will or interest it is doubtful that pleasure or benefit will be derived. Force is inexcusable.

Respect for the individual is important, and some people are naturally very private and abhor any group activity. The picture of a jolly sing-along in a ward for old people is attractive, but remember, to some people such activity is terrible. People who dislike group activities can be encouraged to appreciate private activities. The needs of people such as this can be identified and met.

Suggested Reading

R. Attenborough, **The Attenborough Report: Arts in the Health Service**, *London, Carnegie Trust*, 1985.

H. Butterfield Picard and J.B. Magno, The role of occupational therapy in hospice care, **American Journal of Occupational Therapy**, 36: Sept. 1982, 597–8.

P. Coles, **Art in the NHS**, *London: DHSS*, 1983.

Council for Music in Hospitals Annual Reports, 1983–92.

A. Holland, and K. Nelson-Tigges, The hospice movement – a time for professional action and commitment, **British Journal of Occupational Therapy**, 44: 373–6, 1981.

G. Lord, **The Arts and Disabilities**, *Edinburgh: Macdonald*, 1981.

B. Robb, **Sans everything**, *London: Nelson & Sons*, 1967.

R. Rowden, Music pulled them through, **Nursing Mirror**, 8 Aug. 1984, pp. 32–4.

R. Rowden, Dance for children with hearing impairment, **Sound Barrier**, *RNID Journal*, Spring 1985.

R. Rowden, Will you, won't you join the dance? **Parents' Voice**, *Journal of MENCAP*, Summer 1985.

M.J. Spencer, **The Healing Role of the Arts: A European Perspective**, *New York: Rockefeller Foundation*, 1983.

G.D. Wilson, **The Psychology of Performing Arts**, *Beckenham: Croom Helm*, 1985.

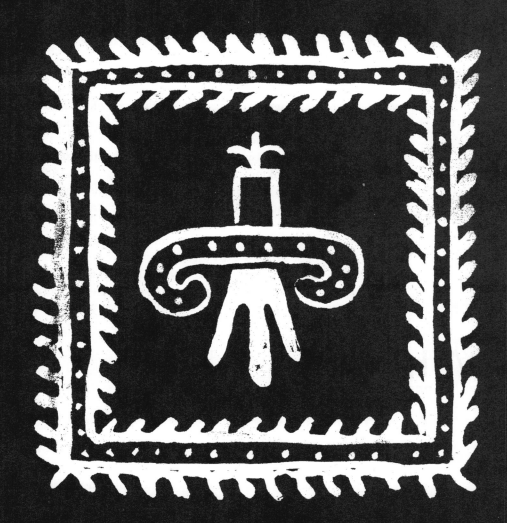

3

ART THERAPY

Camilla Connell and Regan Wright

Long before the written word was part of our heritage art was used to communicate spiritual and psychological truths. It was known in the past that imagery could conduct influences which would penetrate different levels of human consciousness, thus communicating understanding and knowledge, to emotions as well as intellect. It is this wordless process which informs the therapeutic effect experienced when viewing or making art. In the words of Adamson (1984), 'The visual arts are more than a palliative – under the right guidance, they can be a vital form of self-help which allows Nature's healing powers to restore balance and harmony to the troubled mind.'[1]

Although to engage with art can be considered one of the oldest of therapeutic activities, art therapy as a profession is still young. In Britain the term *art therapy* was used in the 1940s, and the first post established in the National Health Service was in a state mental hospital in 1946, but it was not until 1981 that the profession was officially recognised in the Health Service.

What is an Art Therapist?

The description of the British Association of Art Therapists (BAAT) in the Register of 1991 reads:

> Qualified Art Therapists have a considerable understanding of art processes, are proficient in the area of non-verbal communication and are able to provide a trusting and facilitating environment in which patients feel safe to express strong emotions. Their graduate training enables them to work in a variety of settings: Psychiatry, Mental Handicap, Special Education, the Social Services and Prisons. It is important to remember that art therapy is a diverse profession.
>
> Only art therapists who have registered with BAAT can be known to be practising to the standards we, as a professional body uphold.[2]

Research

One of the major criticisms levelled at art therapy by those unconvinced of its effectiveness is the lack of conclusive evidence of results. Research into art therapy in Britain has admittedly been

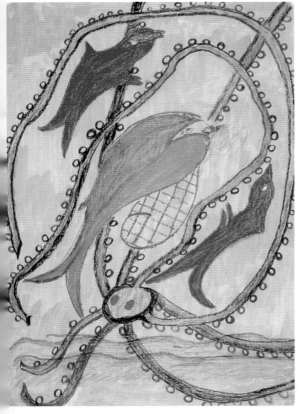

Plate 3.1   Octopus and dolphins

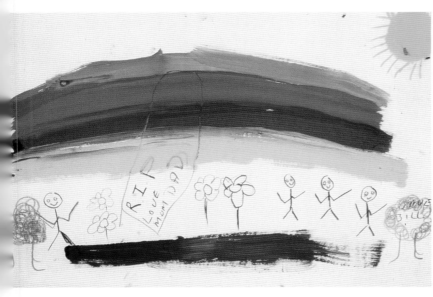

Plate 3.2   R.I.P.

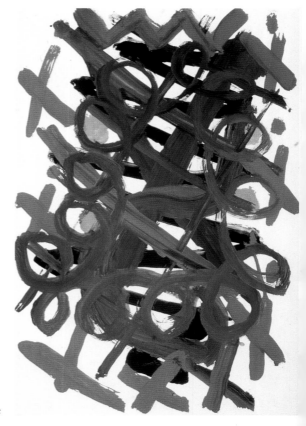

Plate 3.3   Red and black crosses

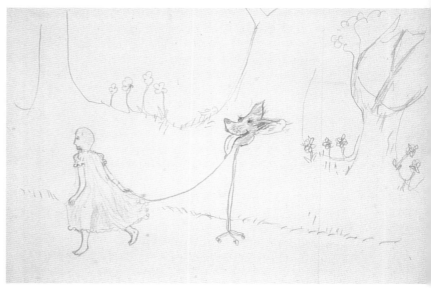

Plate 3.4   Chemotherapy

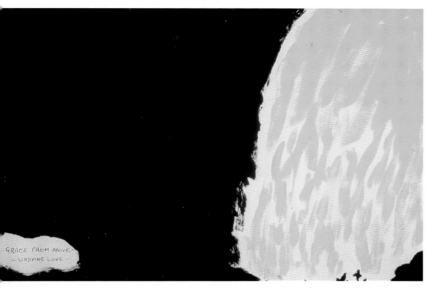

Plate 3.5   Grace from above

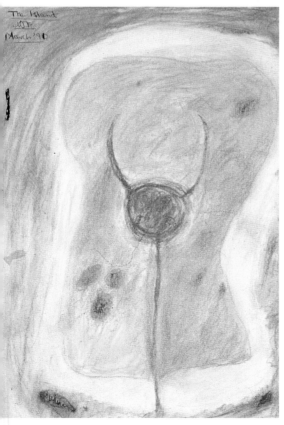

Plate 3.6   The Island

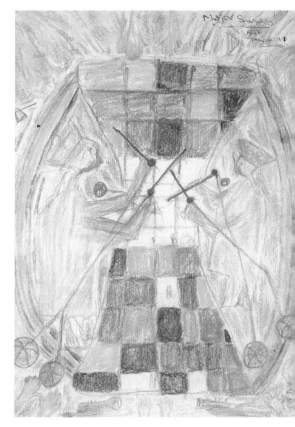

Plate 3.7   Major surgery

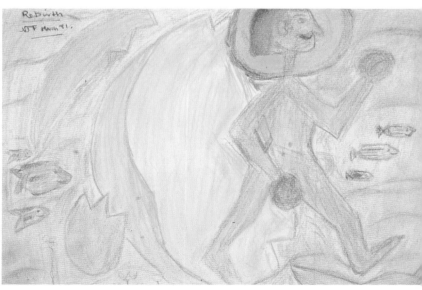

Plate 3.8   Rebirth

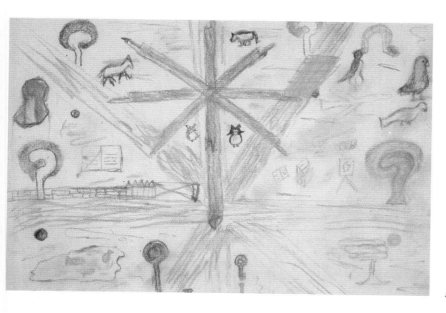

Plate 3.9   Keys and crossroads

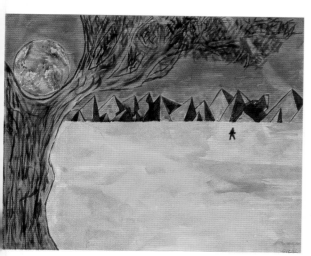

Plate 3.10   Pearl at the bottom of the ocean

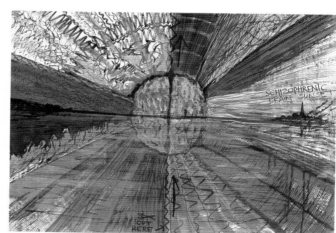

Plate 3.11   Schizophrenic brain sunset

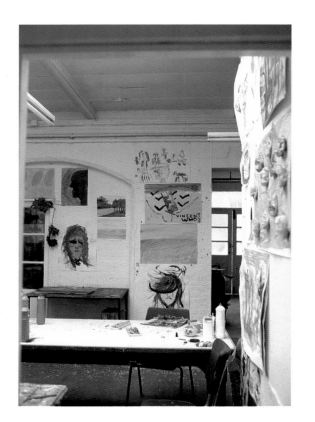

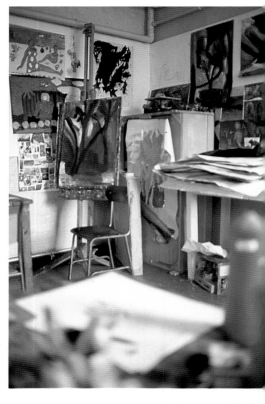

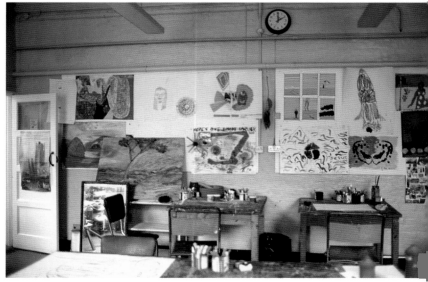

Plate 3.12   Art therapy studios

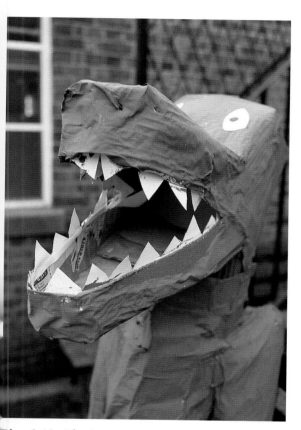

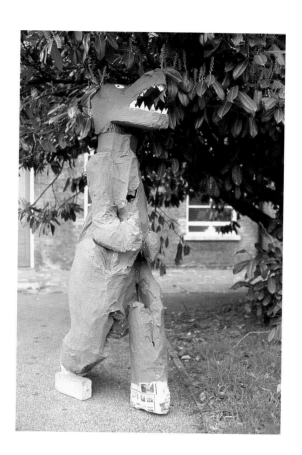

Plate 3.13   The Power Monster

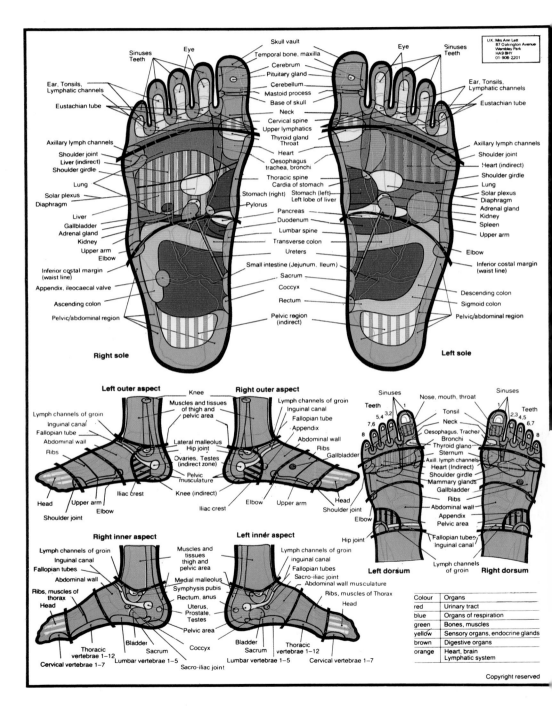

Plate 9.1   Reflex zones of the feet. Reproduced with the permission of Hanne Marquardt.

rather sporadic and unsystematic. Far more work has been done in the USA, particularly in the areas of clinical effectiveness and diagnosis ... It is hard to find conclusive statistical results in art therapy research which are anyway notoriously difficult to achieve.[3]

However, it is always possible to look to the consumer in order to evaluate the processes involved. Feedback from the patient in terms of spontaneous comment occurs quite frequently, and the artwork itself provides evidence of the power of image making which is undeniable.

To give a broad account of art therapy in health care in this chapter would be to understate its place in the different settings within the overall areas of practice. For this reason we have split the chapter into two sections and the accounts given will be descriptions of experience gained in two specific and very different National Health Service hospitals.

Art therapy
in a National Health Service cancer hospital

Art therapy has long been recognised as having a valuable part to play in the treatment of mental illness. This will be considered in the second half of the chapter. Only recently, with the development of interest in complementary therapies in the area of life-threatening illnesses such as cancer, has art therapy found a place there. For a number of years art therapy has been part of the programme for patients attending the Bristol Cancer Help Centre, and increasingly it is now being used in hospices throughout the country. In 1989 the Royal Marsden Hospital was the first NHS cancer hospital to establish an art therapy service as part of its newly opened Marie Curie Rehabilitation Centre.

As with other creative therapies this particular discipline can offer an opportunity for the expression of psychic and emotional needs by non-verbal means, the value of which is irreplaceable for some people when words are inadequate or inappropriate.

Art is able to cut through and transcend the taboos that surround the acceptance of death, and this can be of great therapeutic value for those who are coming to the end of their life and face the imminence of death.[4]

To receive a diagnosis of an illness which poses a threat to our very existence is immediately a shock to most people, particularly if this diagnosis is cancer, the development of which can be so insidious and the outcome unknown. When initial reactions subside, many other concerns may arise and exert a pressure on their bearers whether or not they find that they are conscious of them. Time becomes a unique factor in this illness. Individuals are faced with the fact that life as they know it is finite, and they may experience a need for growth in understanding while there is yet time. In this situation priorities can change and the scale of life's values alters greatly. Throughout the course of the illness, and with such changes as these, it may be difficult for some people to find words to express what it is they need or for what they are searching. Troubling questions can then often be addressed through the non-verbal medium of art, and words will ensue when the images, often symbolic, have been released into a picture. These may enable a communication to take place between different parts of the person's own psyche and also between one person and another. Art therapy is thus ideally suited and can be of great service to individuals trying to understand their situation and needing to improve their quality of life.

The art therapist working in this setting, unlike other uniformed members of staff, does not occupy a clearly defined role. Although not a member of the much-needed medical team upon whom patients feel they depend for their well-being or survival, art therapists can often meet patients on a different ground where these concerns can be aired.

Art therapists have to initiate, offer materials, look, listen and reflect. However, they do not lead the way; they can only accompany. Their most important function is to offer a safe space within which patients feel enabled to experiment and approach the unknown for themselves through image making. This bridge building from surface levels of experience to deeper ones can be what is needed when the ego is finally brought to relinquish its hold and the individual can begin to make contact with another mode of awareness. The importance of this cannot be overestimated for someone facing a life-threatening illness and for whom other forms of intervention, be they physical or psychological, may not facilitate that passage. The creative endeavour can assist this necessary 'healing' step. In the area of cancer care, art therapy can be offered at any stage of illness. It has been found to be particularly valuable during periods of crisis, soon after diagnosis and initial treatment, at times of recurrence and in later illness when it becomes evident that the outlook is not good. Some people who have had difficulty in resolving other psychological issues have found it helpful to come as outpatients to a group session where they are able to paint and work over a longer period than that of the majority of inpatients.

WHO BENEFITS FROM ART THERAPY?

Who would benefit from this type of intervention? Is it for everybody, or only a few? How are such people identified, and can they be readily identified? Is there a process of referral? Addressing these questions in reverse, it is possible to say that formal referrals are not frequent, yet the support of other members of staff in this respect is much appreciated when it occurs.

The reason for this absence of interest in involving art therapists in a multi-disciplinary team is that the potentially deep and significant effect of such an intervention is not well understood. Art therapy is frequently seen as merely offering diversion to a bored or anxious patient. It is not easy to assess instantly if an individual would find such a creative opportunity helpful, with appropriate encouragement, in coping with the present situation. When words are inadequate, people are not necessarily able to reveal their needs or even formulate them for themselves. It is often necessary to form a genuine relationship with a patient, trying to share interests and concerns until a certain trust is established and the patient feels safe enough to venture into the unfamiliar area of 'art'. Nevertheless, artwork is not for all. Some people have strong attitudes about it which seem unshakeable; some have a fear of entering the unknown which inhibits any attempt – and quite understandably; some fear a loss of face, of 'not being able to paint'; and some have a simple absence of interest. The approach of the therapist has to be flexible and imaginative.

ENCOUNTERING ART THERAPY

In a hospital such as the Royal Marsden, patients' length of stay is very variable. For some it may be one or two days, for some six weeks or more. There are also those who are admitted on a regular basis for courses of treatment which are repeated over many months. Duration of involvement with artwork can influence the outcome, but even for those whose contact is brief, much can happen in one session.

Initially, someone may reject any suggestion of working with art materials; indeed, this is often the case. Remarks are made, such as 'I am no good at drawing,' 'I can't paint,' 'I was told I was hopeless at school', 'You couldn't find anyone less artistic than me.' So ways have to be found to quieten fears, engender enthusiasm, and instil the idea that it is not required that a 'good' painting should be forthcoming but that it is possible to enjoy the process for its own sake and allow oneself to experiment and explore without fear of the results. Of course, to someone faced with a blank sheet of paper and no 'inspiration', this is easier said than done. It is quite an heroic leap for some people to start painting. Others will fall on the materials with delight and enthusiasm, saying that they have never had time to try this sort of thing before, or that they used to enjoy art, but it was a very long time ago, and so on.

There are many different responses, and the therapist has to accommodate them all, trying to find the best way to enable the patients to allow themselves to engage with the materials. These may be presented and arranged so as to be as conducive as possible to experimentation. A selection of crayons offered should be of good quality and different characteristics: water soluble, charcoal-textured, soft wax crayons or felt-tip pens. These all offer a slightly different experience in use and in the effect they produce. There are varieties of coloured tissue papers which can be cut, torn and stuck for a collage. This is often a good starting point for some who may be afraid of using paint, as it helps them to surmount the first hurdle of 'not being able to paint'. Clay too should be available. Paints are offered in transparent, lidded plastic pots so the colours are visible, and these should be arranged in shallow plastic trays in sets of ten to twelve with a jam jar for water and sets of brushes of varying sizes, from house painting size down to very fine and small. In this way, patients have a choice and may feel encouraged to try.

THE GROUP NOTEBOOK

One of the most useful and rewarding tools which has developed in this setting over the past two years is a group notebook. This provides a means for otherwise isolated patients to communicate with one another. Borrowing the title *Memories, Dreams, Reflections* from Jung,[5] it covers most themes likely to be prevalent in the experience of hospitalised patients with cancer. This notebook is an A4 loose-leaf binder. The sheets of work are inserted into clear plastic envelopes with perforations for the rings. These protect and enhance the appearance of the work, enabling it to be handled frequently without damage. At present there are about fifty pages depicting a wide range of experience and comment. This is like a group notebook as it offers some of the benefits derived from cancer support groups. Since many patients are admitted for short periods, ongoing groups do not seem to be a practical possibility for many, yet at the critical periods of hospitalisation a recognition that they are not alone in their difficulties can be of comfort. In comparing themselves with others through the artwork in the book, patients can gain a perspective about their own emotional reactions. As in a group, self-worth is enhanced in the receiving and giving of support through art and written work. Hope and understanding can be shared even when the worst fears and losses are depicted.

This notebook often serves a valuable purpose as the focus of an opening conversation between patient and therapist. By going through it together, it is possible to amplify what is on the page by recalling remarks that were made when the work was done, if appropriate. Often responses are readily forthcoming from the patients who identify with, or react to the picture in front of them. Sometimes three or four patients will gather round and look together, exchanging comments. Many people are apprehensive about drawing and painting, so this viewing serves to reassure them that most people are not 'talented' and that it is quite acceptable to make very simple renderings of any topic they wish, or even to doodle. If encouraged by what they have seen, patients who wish to 'have a go' are offered an A4 pad and materials of their choice. If they make something that they feel they would like to contribute to the note book they are told that it will be much valued and seen by many people. Indeed this is so, and looking through it over and over again with patients one sees what an extraordinary human testimony it is.

THE BENEFITS OF ART THERAPY

In what way can art in therapy alleviate or enlighten the situation of someone with cancer? The artwork itself can indicate how powerful the effect can be, but what other evidence is there? It is difficult to evaluate art therapy scientifically, but in addition to the work done there are many verbal comments made by patients which are some indication of how the process is experienced: 'I am sorry I said so much, but I feel better for it,' was the remark of one woman after a group meeting. 'It was good to have a brush in my hand and paint through the pain' – from a woman having recently undergone a mastectomy. 'It is so busy everywhere, the art therapy room seems quite different, cut off from the rest, like an island of peace,' was another unsolicited remark. 'I found I didn't worry about what anyone else thought, I was painting just for myself and could enjoy it very much;' 'It is good to release these feelings, it is so surprising what comes up. I can be like this away from home,' were two more comments.

An example showing the enjoyment and liberation to be obtained by painting is illustrated by an elderly unmarried lady who was convinced that drawing and painting were not 'her thing' and quite beyond her. She was in the ward for many weeks and she had talked about her interests in archaeology, gardening and embroidery. One day she was shown some pictures of Minoan wall paintings and had it suggested to her that she might like to make a design for her embroidery. This was acceptable and she worked on her design for five weeks. On one occasion this reluctant lady was so keen to get to the art session that she fell out of her wheelchair. The drawing gave her much pleasure and she was delighted with her achievement; eventually it was framed for her. Although she became gradually more incapacitated, a friendly contact was maintained and she liked having collages made for her while she visualised and described their content in detail (Plate 3.1).

In the unfamiliar surroundings of a hospital, and having to cope with their illness, many people feel isolated, and painting becomes a means of communication. Most people have no tuition in painting or drawing, but even the simplest attempts will elicit a response from others, giving the makers respite from their feelings of isolation. One such example is the work of a young man of twenty-eight experiencing a recurrence of a brain tumour which he knew was inoperable. Quite unaccustomed to artwork, he began by painting some simple stripes across the paper, but then abandoning the brush and taking up a pencil, depicted his own funeral with his family and friends standing round. Having described this he simply said that he was sorry but that was how he felt. He had been enabled, by the drawing, to speak of what was uppermost in his mind but for which no words seemed appropriate (Plate 3.2).

Emotional conflicts surrounding the concern for a diseased body are often concealed in order to protect the conscious mind from pain. To force a recognition of these issues may either traumatise or increase denial, but spontaneous picture making can allow the unconscious level to emerge, inviting acknowledgement but not demanding it. Thus the image challenges the protective mechanisms but does not assault them. At first K felt apprehensive about using paint, so she was offered some coloured tissue paper and glue in order to make a collage of what she decided would be a Japanese sun. A few days later K proudly showed what she had done. Her 'sun' had turned into a 'breast' and she had been delighted at the interest her surgeon had shown in her work with the comments he had made. He had said that he thought a cockade was a medal for gallantry and that a purple triangle was her inverted nipple and the area where the disease had been. It seemed that K was trying to come to terms with her condition when she remarked that breasts were frivolous things as well as important things.

At all stages of illness – be it diagnosis, recurrence, or later, with the loss of independence and physical and psychological functioning – feelings such as shock, confusion, anger and fear may arise. Through painting these feelings can be expressed without fear of remorse or retribution. The artwork can permit a *cri de coeur* to be heard which might never otherwise find a voice. There is often a need for some form of cathartic release even in very ill people and it is not possible to judge someone's psychological state from their outward appearance. This was shown very clearly when L was approached just for a short conversation. She seemed happy to recall her past as a teacher and talked at length. An awareness of how she must be feeling was expressed and she was shown a few paints, whereupon she said that she would like to have 'a splash' after all. The materials were set up for her in the position in which she was half lying, half sitting. Therapist and other patients nearby who were aware of how ill she was were amazed to see her rapidly gather her energy as she applied paint to paper with increasingly confident movements, until after a quarter of an hour she had made a bold and beautiful painting of flowers in a vase. Then asking for another sheet of paper she attacked it, covering it with red and black crosses and swirling circles, surmounted by what looked like a crown. Lying back L exclaimed 'Phew, that's better!' Then she explained that she had started gently just painting the flowers, then the vase to give it a firm base and finally putting black on the tips of the flowers to 'balance it'. With the second painting she felt different, she said, scrabbling on the paper with her fingers in frustration as she spoke. 'I really had to beat this thing and felt very angry. Now I feel much better for it and just want to sit.' The next day L was too weak to speak and three days later she died. She had apparently needed this one and only opportunity to release these feelings. In this brief encounter there was no time for any formulation of therapeutic aims; art therapy could just offer a vehicle for the outpouring of a human spirit as it went on its way (Plate 3.3).

Some people may react with fear and resentment towards the hospital and treatments they are having to undergo. Feelings of impotence in the face of the suffering they endure can also arise. Relief is sometimes found through drawing or painting where these feelings can be openly expressed and thus somewhat neutralised without violence or the risk of damaging relationships. Such feelings towards chemotherapy were well expressed by a young student in a drawing of a hairless woman patient going for a walk taking with her on a lead her dog, or is it a wolf? But this animal is disembodied and one sees that it is but a head, fixed to a drip stand, the tongue representing the bottle containing the aggressive chemotherapy drug. Through this drawing the patient has very powerfully communicated her feelings about her treatment (Plate 3.4).

On the other hand, patients will often enjoy depicting things in their lives which are important to them, reminding them of home or of times past, all of which they miss in the hospital environment. Many examples exist, but a picture made by a middle-aged farmer's wife with advanced lung cancer, who is now reflecting sadly on the things she was able to do in the year before she became too ill, was typical. She told the small art group of the wild year she had had with her husband when she knew she had cancer but before it imposed limitations on her activities, and how she had loved to climb the hill behind their house and fly a kite in the wind.

Artwork can display concerns on different psychological levels. Frequently there appears an expression of, or a search for, the impulses of love, faith and hope. It does seem that very often there are no words available or adequate for feelings of this nature. Through their suffering and knowledge of their illness people are often brought to a point where these sentiments take on a great importance and the wordless process of image making can allow them to surface and be communicated to the patients themselves and to others. To assist this to happen, the therapist should already have gained the trust of the patients and then try to impart an impression of openness and receptivity to them so that the patients feel that they are held in a situation that is safe enough for whatever in them is seeking to appear through imagery, to do so. In the example illustrated in Plate 3.5, an elderly woman patient with advanced illness was anxious to communicate a vision she felt she had received during the night. She entitled it 'Grace from Above, Undying Love'. She made one version for the art therapist and one for the chaplain who had been visiting her. It gave her meaning to be able to present this to the therapist and discuss it with her.

The therapist should try to make more and more space for the patient to speak because, as Winnicott says, 'It is not the moment of my clever interpretation that is significant'.[6] The value in art for patients is when they come to their *own* understanding. The role of the therapist is as an attendant while the patients traverse this threshold for themselves.

Some patients will use art quite deliberately as a way of coping with their situations or of stretching their understanding and for re-evaluating their lives, questioning where necessary the direction in which they should go. To have reached this stage a patient will have taken a quite significant step in acknowledging their illness and its possible outcome. There do not seem to be a great number of people who are able to let themselves be so open to their predicament, but for those who are, the process of picture making can be a valuable part in their becoming more whole.

One such young man, N, was in hospital for the first time, newly diagnosed and undergoing surgery for cancer in his bladder. During his stay he made what he called a diary of his experience. He had obtained some charcoal crayons and paper from another patient. When the therapist first met N, he had already started work, having completed the first two of a series of pictures which were to depict a very revealing pattern of thought and feeling. Although he did not use many words in these drawings he did give them titles and then took great delight in getting the therapist to try to describe what she thought he was trying to say through them. The therapist was reluctant to describe N's ideas for him, and he was encouraged to describe in considerable detail each drawing as it appeared.

'The Island'

N said that this image arose partly from an impression he had retained from passing over islands in a plane, but that it also represented his torso. The pond in the centre of the island was his bladder, which, as can be seen, is complete with ureters and urethra, and the green fishes inside the bladder were consuming his cancer cells (Plate 3.6).

'The Family Tree'

N described this picture as showing his parents as two large trees in the foreground, while he and his brother are behind, represented by two smaller trees. Roots and branches are intertwined, forming at the same time a chalice in the branches which represents the sacrament of marriage between the parent trees. It also reminded him of the sands of time, for them, for him, or for both. He also said that repeated images of three encircled plants spoke of his closeness to his parents.

'Major Surgery'

In the third drawing, which is entitled 'Major Surgery', N described how two surgeons with wool and needles are 'knitting' him back to health in the form of a patchwork quilt. These surgeons also become conductors of music, surrounded by healing hands and musical instruments. The rainbows represent healing or spiritual forces (Plate 3.7).

'Symbolic Fruit'

'Symbolic Fruit' is the title of a drawing of a richly coloured mango and a banana hanging from the same slender stalk. N had said that the picture described how heavy he had felt 'down there' after his operation.

'Rebirth'

In a watery environment a man in red boxing gloves is breaking out of a golden eggshell and striding out of the picture. N thought that the halo indicated a sort of new spiritual awareness. He said that he was concerned that the smile on his face could seem fixed and meaningless, but in fact he felt it as positive. Again the healing fish appear (Plate 3.8).

'Crossroads'

There are two crosses in this picture, each with seven branches; maybe they are on different planes. Birds, keys and keyholes, small animals, and again the healing fishes are all part of this complex picture (Plate 3.9.).

This is an interesting series of drawings because it describes very fully the inner processes undergone during the episode of this young man's illness. The diagnosis immediately brought N to the point of re-evaluating all aspects of his life: firstly and most directly, his body, seen in isolation as an island and with a wish for healing forces to be at work, indicated by the presence of the fishes; secondly, his need for and appreciation of his family. He recognises a sacred quality to this relationship, but also that it is subject to the sands of passing time and is not endless. All the encircled triple images seem to suggest a protective quality that his family life offers him. Then comes his multi-faceted body entrusted to surgeons surrounded by the healing forces of light, sound and hands. Or maybe they are bridging a gap in his life-span and restoring the continuity that seemed to be broken by illness? Again, post-operatively, his body reclaims his attention, the 'fruit' of his manhood is a focus of his awareness and concern. This vulnerability is then replaced by a new spirit of regeneration. One is reminded of the golden egg from which Brahma burst forth in Hindu tradition. Here is

N, mind over body; he is determined to overcome his illness but not without recognising in the final drawing, 'Crossroads', that there were question marks as to the direction his life should now take. Embodied in trees they seem living questions; doubled, they form keys. It seems that N felt himself at a new axis derived from an older underlying one. Through suffering his orientation might change; struggle and choice seem to offer themselves to him – a new perspective through illness on an existence which had previously gone unquestioned.

SUMMARY

Art therapy is beginning to be recognised as having a part to play in the management of life-threatening illness. This discipline should be incorporated within the existing medical model and should not be viewed merely as a light-weight occupational pastime. Kearney, a contemporary advocate for the inclusion of therapists with skills such as art therapy in the multi-disciplinary team says:

> We need to recognise that they are not just diversional therapies, optional extras or therapeutic luxuries which belong to the periphery of the palliative care programme but important healing skills which should have a place at the centre of the palliative care approach. From one perspective they might be seen as a contemporary expression of the medieval 'ars moriendi' (art of dying) as the crossing of the boundary line from the surface level to the deep is experienced by the ego as a sort of death. If, on the other hand, one looks at them in the context of the personal transformation, new birth or healing they may lead to, they might be seen as an interesting variant of 'midwifery skills'! However the threshold crossing skills are viewed, they may be as important to the process of healing as morphine is to pain control.[7]

Art therapy
in mental health

The second part of this chapter introduces art therapy in a large psychiatric hospital which offers treatments for adults with all types of mental illness.

The buildings vary from those designed as institutions in early Victorian days to some of very recent design where the site is being condensed and streamlined according to current NHS policy.

Art therapy has been available here since 1966, which reflects the fact that psychiatry is the field where it was first established, and where it is still mainly used. As a profession it has developed considerably. The emphasis has moved from the provision of a diversionary skills-orientated context to one which attempts to develop self-awareness and insight, and the use of creativity as a positive and very personal resource. In this way a balance is also explored between the necessary intervention of medical care and the encouragement of the clients' own ability to discover healthy ways of changing and adapting to their difficulties. It is important to note that clients, when discussing art therapy, often stress that it is the process they go through which provides the insight, not simply the end product. This is highlighted in the commentaries to the illustrations which follow.

'Pearl at the Bottom of the Ocean'

This picture (Plate 3.10) was painted by a client admitted in the mid-1970s with an acute drink problem. This involved 'black-out' periods which were thought to be related to alcohol abuse. However, it soon became clear that he was suffering from a deep underlying depression, and the black-outs were part of his unconscious attempt to avoid his despair. At first he avoided all verbal communication, having become isolated and easily threatened by other people. However, he found pictures a good way to express his internal conflict. As often happens when art therapy is working well, the pictures poured out without conscious intention or pre-set ideas. When the pictures were finished, and as he gained confidence, he began to apply his intelligence to try to understand what he had painted. The therapist's part in this process is to listen to any explanation of how the image has occurred; to ask questions until the subject is fully understood, and then to ask more questions until the artist's attitude to the work is clear. These questions must be put carefully so that they do not intrude, and nor should they suggest a particular line of thought. The intention is to be able to empathise with the experience, but also to function as someone on the outside who can bring an objective view to the situation, and who can also contain or 'hold' some of the feelings for a while, if they are too painful for the client. The therapist is someone who is aware of the meaning of making images, and who can help to make links between conscious and unconscious material, and intellectual and emotional experience.

In this particular picture it is possible to see that the artist has reached a clear understanding of his emotional situation. He is isolated in an arid land of his own, and must find a way back to the world. It contains all the power and energy that this understanding has released, but it also suggests some of the uncertainty and fear which cannot be avoided in this sort of personal process.

This emphasis on self-discovery and self-reliance, with the patient or clients having increased responsibility for finding ways of understanding their condition, learning to tolerate their confusion and despair, and to look for solutions, has steadily developed in psychiatry. Much attention has been payed to how to facilitate this process, which is one of the reasons why creative therapies have been encouraged.

Most people who experience some form of mental illness see themselves, at times, as 'outsiders' who cannot cope with society. They may be highly critical of social convention, or they may feel desperately inadequate and rejected, or something in between these two extremes, but they do not feel part of a reasonably consistent lifestyle to which they feel others belong. One definition of people who have become mentally ill is that they have been 'forced to compromise too much too soon.' This last sentence is a paraphrase of theories developed by the psychiatrist R.D. Laing who explored the conflicts involved in an individual's survival in society, amongst other issues. This compromise has left them with a damaged sense of self which cannot sustain the pressures of existence and coexistence. Medication is enormously important in relieving some of the intolerable symptoms and stress, and provides some stability for patients with long-term conditions. Understanding the chemicals involved with brain dysfunction develops all the time, and so drug treatment has become very much more effective with far fewer destructive side effects. However, it is recognised that there must also be work towards rebuilding the damaged personality. Good medication will often allow this potential development which would otherwise be impossible.

Therapy should be an assertively open-ended situation in which patients or clients have the maximum opportunity to find their own direction and therefore begin to build self-awareness and insight on their own terms. It is no longer important to make the 'right' interpretations, but instead to offer suggestions, provide alternative ways of looking at things, to challenge assumptions, and generally to attempt to provide a very active feedback and response. This provides understanding of the client's position, and how it came about, and a chance to help find ways forward, and ways of changing by focusing on the client's own resources. In this way, 'getting better' should become a concept that has some personal reality related to the client's sense of what is appropriate, rather than, as sometimes occurs, an unreal fantasy which is really an unconscious resistance to change, mostly through fear.

To do this well, it is important to be aware of psychoanalytic theory, to be informed about the work of major psychologists and psychotherapists and to be aware of fundamental mental processes and the way in which behaviour is structured. Art therapists do not usually follow one particular school of thought, but instead employ a range of different ideas from leading psychoanalysts. This has been called the 'cook-book' approach.

From pre-history onwards human beings have used image making as an important feature in the social structure. We have always valued this way of defining our experience, identifying our hopes and fears, and using colour and shape as a successful way of communicating which not only allows contacts which are verbal events through spontaneous self-expression, but which can also represent our feelings more successfully than words. This is because the process of translating an idea into metaphor and symbolism is very personal and so will emphasise each individuals' particular identity. Once objectified into an image, the emotional material can become much more accessible to reason and understanding.

If one separates the idea of image making from technical skill and professional sophistication, one can see it as a universal process whereby individuals can find their own particular language of self-expression. It is a way of introducing someone to unconscious material in a fairly gentle manner, which should always leave the artist feeling reasonably in control since he or she dictates the content of the work, and can decide on the level of discussion about it. In this way a bridge between isolated individuals and the people surrounding them can be built, not by encouraging a conformist approach but by concentrating on understanding exactly what each person feels. In this way it is hoped that a comfortable working compromise can be reached between the need of the individual and the realities of society. It is important to stress this factor, because most people suffering from a form of mental illness are very aware of the conflict between, as they see it, becoming ostracised by the sense of not being able to fit in, or the pressure to subdue their own needs and take on a passive and unacceptable role. When such sufferers are in this position, other people are perceived subjectively as being powerful and in control, and so appear as very frightening. This can then generate the paranoid and angry state of mind which helps to make communication difficult.

'Schizophrenic Brain Sunset'

This is a beautiful but angry painting to explain what schizophrenia is like (Plate 3.11). The negative power of the situation is very clear. The artist has much strength and energy, but in general it is hard for him to translate these attributes into something he can use. This person is very intelligent but, as a condition of this illness he has trouble with linking his intellect with his emotions so that they tend to function separately with a very disabling result. However, he manages to combine thinking and feeling quite successfully in this picture, which was an important achievement for him in the process of learning something about how to deal with the effect of his illness.

Art therapy can be summed up by a quotation from a patient: 'I have learnt that my pictures are never wrong'.

Another issue, so far not touched on, but which is very important, relates to the multi-cultural society we live in. We must recognise and learn about the differences with which other individuals view the use of art. There is much positive research in this field, and more needs to be done. As a team we are now being asked to do much more with people from minority ethnic groups, which is a fascinating and complex development.

THE SERVICE OFFERED

What is it like being an art therapist? In this psychiatric hospital there is a team of three and a department consisting of two large studios and an office (Plate 3.12). Every morning there are 'open sessions' or workshops in the studios, and these are available to individually referred inpatients and outpatients. In fact, two-thirds of the people who use these sessions are outpatients, which is in line with the move away from institutional care. There are also art therapy groups in areas of specialist care. Currently, these involve the elderly, the alcohol abuse service, long-stay rehabilitation clients and the intense psychotherapy programme.

There are also sessions in the local mental health resource centres (or MHRC). These are based in the community, and are intended to provide a very varied and flexible treatment programme for anyone experiencing psychiatric problems. Art therapy is one of the available para-medical specialisms, and as such has become a much more accepted and established part of treatment available in the NHS. The problem now is that there is often a conflict between the clinical needs of a developing service, and the financial pressures due to a general shortage of funds.

One of the most noticeable pieces of work in the art department is a large papier-mâché animal, vaguely like a dinosaur (Plate 3.13). This is referred to as the 'power monster'. It was made by a young man at the end of his treatment programme. He had problems related to his family background which had left him clinically depressed, passive-angry and defeated. His attitude was that he could not find any confidence in himself and therefore no motivation to change. He was still over-dependent on his family, but was also desperate to separate from them, and this ambivalence made it very difficult for him to move forward. He had to do much hard work to begin to confront these problems, and to find ways of making them more tolerable. It became clear that one of the underlying features of his passivity was an unconscious fear of his own power and energy because, in the course of his childhood, these passive resources had got confused with his anger and frustration and so had come to seem dangerous. The power monster was built to establish a contact with these long-suppressed characteristics, so that he could begin to sort out what was positive and what was negative in this part of himself.

Members of the department got quite involved in the process of making this sculpture. There was a time when the body of the monster began to collapse and many jokes (some of them very crass) were made as suggestions about how it might be made to stand up. In fact, a lot of art therapy work involves wit and humour as well as every other combination of emotions that one can think of. Some of the work is ugly; most of it is interesting in one way or another; occasionally it is beautiful. It is almost always very accessible to the viewer. Once the basic philosophy is understood, everyone can look at the work and understand something of what the artist has experienced and wishes to communicate. It can be seen that what someone who is ill is having to cope with is not so different from what we all have to deal with, but perhaps in a much more extreme form.

Therapists need to keep open minds both in terms of keeping up with current research and developments in the field, and also in listening to what the clients have to say. They do not, like members of some other professions, have a very clear philosophical model to work with, preferring to use ideas from all sorts of different sources. This has advantages and disadvantages. This can be defined in terms of the emphasis on the individual and the flexibility of approach. It can also be quite a strain to continue to work in a way that constantly demands a varied approach. There are 'methods of work' practices to combat this problem for therapists and clients. Great attention is paid to organising boundaries to work practice. This relates to the way the sessions are structured in terms of expectations, time limits and so on. It also relates to the kind of relationships therapists have with clients. These must all be clear in order to provide an effective 'container' environment which allows people to feel safe to express their personal conflicts.

Therapists also need to be clear about their own needs, and to learn about the pitfalls of their unconscious omnipotence which leads them to expect more of their clients and themselves than is healthy. There are other situations, such as supervision groups on sessions, which are intended to give therapists somewhere to take their professional problems and pressures and to make sure that they continue to function as they should.

Conclusion

For readers who consider that this type of work could be beneficial for patients in their care, the obvious question is, how to conduct an activity of this nature and how to begin. Is it enough to offer art materials and encourage a patient to use them? Simple as it seems, the power of image making should never be underestimated. On one level it would appear to offer a harmless and pleasant form of entertainment. However, images do not arise solely from the logical part of the mind. In fact, under pressure, they are more likely to spring from much deeper emotional levels, over which we do not have conscious control. Material which may emerge can have a powerful and sometimes disturbing effect on patients and therapists. It is important, therefore, that therapists should be able to contain emotional situations that arise safely, and 'establish a therapeutic frame in which the image can be allowed its own authority, without overwhelming the client with its message, but also without being stripped of its iconological power'.[8] Frequently pictures appear depicting despair, frustration, shock, cynicism, uncertainty, fear, muddle and confusion, loss and sadness. These need to be allowed to stand and to be acknowledged. Yet, having expressed such feelings in a drawing or painting, the maker often experiences relief from the pressure they were exerting.

The therapist, however, may find difficulty in remembering that the patient's feelings are not his or her feelings and may therefore unwittingly become identified with them. Supervision by someone with psychotherapy training is therefore advisable for any therapist engaging in this work. Reflection on the way in which the therapy is going allows the therapist to regain objectivity in relation to the patient, and also to acknowledge personal issues that may intrude into professional activity. There is a tendency in all of us to try and make terrible situations better. It requires help to resist the need to rescue people from their distress, thereby devaluing it. Encounters with the image-making process cannot be undertaken casually. Powerful responses are evoked. There are risks therefore for both patient and therapist, but also rewarding challenges.

References

1 E. Adamson, **Art as Healing**, *Boston: Coventure*, 1984.

2 British Association of Art Therapists Register, 1991.

3 T. Dalley, (ed.) **Art as Therapy**, *London: Tavistock* 1984.

4 Ibid.

5 C.G. Jung, **Memories, Dreams, Reflections**, *London: Routledge & Kegan Paul*, 1963.

6 D.W. Winnicott, **Playing and Reality**, *London: Tavistock/Penguin Books*, 1971.

7 M. Kearney, Palliative medicine, just another speciality? **Palliative Medicine**, 6(1): 39–46, 1992.

8 M. Edwards, Jungian analytic art therapy, in A.J. Rubin *et al.* **Approaches to Art Therapy**, *New York: Brunner/Mazel*. 1987.

Further Reading

C. Case and T. Dalley, **The Handbook of Art Therapy**, *London: Routledge,* 1992.

C. Connell, Art therapy as part of a palliative care programme, **Palliative Medicine**, 6(1): 18, 1992.

T. Dalley, C. Case, J. Schaverien, F. Weir, P. Nowell-Hall, D. Halliday and D. Waller, **Images of Art Therapy**, *London: Tavistock*, 1987.

R.D. Laing, **The Divided Self**, *Harmondsworth, Penguin*, 1969.

J.A. Rubin, **The Art of Art Therapy**, *New York: Brunner/Mazel*, 1984.

J. Schaverien, **The Revealing Image, Analytical Art Psychotherapy in Theory and Practice**, *London: Routledge,* 1992.

M. Thomson, **On Art and Therapy – An Exploration**, *London: Virago Press*, 1989.

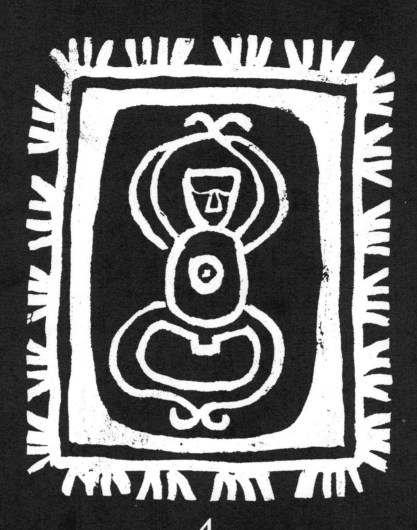

4

RELAXATION AND VISUALISATION

Lynne Ryman

Relaxation and visualisation are two distinct yet vital components of a therapy which allows negative and unhealthy states of mind to be overcome and exchanged for positive, healthy ones.

The role of relaxation in this process is primarily to bring the mind of the participant to a state of balance, quietude and peace, free of negativity. The role of visualisation is to use this balanced state to bring about any changes which a client desires to make. Thus relaxation and visualisation may be seen as working hand in glove when someone wants to become well again, stay well, lose weight, stop smoking and so on.

Relaxation and visualisation are a

> 'planned structured activity in order to gain that elusive quality peace of mind'. Inherent in this state of peace is the ability to control and mitigate levels of tension, worry and anxiety common to us all. It is well . . . documented that too much stress . . . interferes with a person's well-being and ability to enjoy life and if tension is experienced unrelentingly for a long period of time it has . . . a depressing effect on the immune system, leading to . . . ill-health and disease. Human beings are not just physical entities. We consist of physical, emotional, mental and spiritual 'bodies'. For total health and well-being these bodies should be in a state of perfect balance. Disease results when they are not . . .
>
> Relaxation and visualisation are one way in which to regain a healthy, harmonious, whole human being as it provides a necessary and healing break in the daily routine for total relaxation of body, mind and spirit and consequent reaffirmation of homeostasis. It is in this latter state that the body heals itself by lifting those who need it out of despondency into harmony and those who are hyperactive into calmness.[1]

Historical
context

One of the first modern techniques developed specifically for reducing stress was 'progressive relaxation'.[2] Since 1908 Jacobson has been a proponent of this method, and contends that anxiety and relaxation are mutually exclusive because the relaxation of muscles spreads to encompass the entire being.[3] In progressive relaxation the person tenses and then relaxes successive muscle groups. Attention is focused on discriminating between the feelings experienced when the muscle is relaxed compared to when it is tense. Jacobson's procedure entails learning to relax 218 different muscle groups and consequently the technique may take a long time to master.

The 'Relaxation Response' elicited by Benson in 1974 is extremely simple, requiring four essential elements: (1) a quiet environment; (2) a word or phrase repeated over and over again; (3) the adoption of a passive attitude; (4) a comfortable position. The practice of these four elements should result in enhanced well-being.[4]

Visualisation – the ability to use mental imaging to relieve or prevent disease – has existed from earliest times. Shamans or witch doctors in America and Africa used such techniques, as did most early Oriental therapies. From the times of ancient Greece until the Middle Ages it is said to have had great influence and possibly to have provided the origins of Western medicine.[5]

Relaxation and visualisation methods are now being tried and tested throughout the world. Below are just a few examples:

At Bunkyo University in Tokyo studies were done on the degree of acceptance of relaxation and body image reorganisation. These indicated that willingness to apply oneself to the relaxation technique is indispensable for the required change.[6]

Ainslie Meares, an authority on relaxation and visualisation methods, from Australia, travelled the world over a period of years to find a panacea for pain, and subsequently wrote about his experiences.[7] His thesis was to learn as much as he could of the way in which the mind can control the body. He was aware that Eastern mystics are reputed to be able to control pain by meditation and yoga practices. In an article some years ago,[8] Meares discussed differing forms of meditation and relaxation used and reported on a particular technique that he found to be extremely effective in some cases of cancer.

In Canada, it seems, relaxation and visualisation are being applied as one of the strategies in child and youth counselling.[9]

A more unusual example, perhaps, of the use of relaxation is to be found at the Mogilev Works in Russia amongst the 'Stroi maschina' workers in an engineering plant where rooms have been set aside for relaxation.[10] Relaxation was found markedly to reduce the high fatigue levels felt at the end of the shift and also to bring about a considerable reduction of the levels of irritation felt at work and disturbed sleep patterns. Similar research at the Volga motor car works demonstrated a similar pattern.

An interesting development is being attempted in South Africa's Groote Schuur Hospital in Cape Town. Strenuous efforts are being made to set up a Nurse Specialist post to include relaxation and visualisation in its remit. The battle is uphill due, as always, to financial stringencies.[11]

Current
usage

Not only does relaxation help to mitigate levels of stress and mental tension, but, if practised on a regular basis, it can strengthen the immune system, thereby rendering people less susceptible to disease.

In America, where the use of relaxation techniques is quite common, many hospitals teach their patients a programme of relaxation as an integral part of their treatment. Indeed, relaxation can be learnt from a hospital bed just by watching a television broadcast specially devised for the purpose. Health-care workers view relaxation used in this way as enabling patients to help with their own healing.[12]

However, cardiologists have been slow to use such techniques, being unable to believe that stress has much to do with heart disease even though a national health report back in 1984 recommended its use (amongst other things) as a first line of therapy for mild hypertension. Relaxation therapy is now used extensively in the remedial care of heart attack.[13] In Britain, a report in 1985 in the *British Medical Journal*[14] showed that patients who learned to relax maintained an appreciable reduction in their blood pressure and continued to do so for some years.

Relaxation methods are also being used successfully in bringing under control chronic severe pain (whatever its cause), thereby increasing manifoldly patients' ability to enjoy a reasonable quality of life.[15]

These techniques have also been found useful in the management of side effects in procedures such as kidney dialysis and in gastro-intestinal problems like irritable bowel syndrome, and in insomnia and emphysema. Patients undergoing chemotherapy as part of their cancer treatment can use relaxation and visualisation to aid their ability to cope with their treatment, lessen harmful side effects and increase its efficacy.[16]

Relaxation

PROGRESSIVE MUSCLE RELAXATION

Progressive muscle relaxation (pmr) was originated by Jacobson as a result of the realisation that without it people have no means of personal energy conservation.

Pmr is based on the premise that the body responds to emotionally and physically disturbing thoughts and happenings with increased muscle tension. This tension increases the person's experience of anxiety and pain, further increasing muscle tension, thus setting up a vicious circle. It is impossible to be tense and relaxed at the same time. Therefore systematically relaxing the major muscle groups of the body is found to decrease physiological tension; this in turn decreases perceived anxiety and pain.[17]

Using electrical measurements (the integrating neurovoltmeter), Jacobson found that if a person relaxed the external muscles sufficiently – those under his or her (conscious) control – symptoms from excessive internal muscular tension subside.

It is suggested that daily practice (techniques are discussed later) is of great importance for anyone committed to cultivating relaxation. It is necessary to learn to recognise the sensation of tenseness, thereby establishing where and when the tension is present, so that the condition may be counteracted if excessive. Eventually, through regular practice of this technique, relaxation can proceed automatically with little conscious attention.

DEEP BREATHING

Hypoxia (lack of oxygen) is associated with anxiety, irritability, depression, muscle tension and fatigue. Systematic deep breathing can improve oxygenation, leading to a deeply relaxed state, feelings of calm, and an improved ability to cope with stress.[18]

Deep breathing counteracts these anxiety states when carried out on a regular basis. Most therapists use deep breathing as an integral part of their teaching methods.

RESPONSE TO STRESS

The hypothesis is that just as we have an inborn or natural response to flight or fight, each of us possesses a protective and innate mechanism against too much stress which allows us to turn off harmful bodily effects. This response is characterised by decreased heart rate, lowered metabolism, decrease in the rate of breathing and slower brain waves, thus returning the body to a healthier balance. This state is known as the 'Relaxation Response'.[19]

Benson, who first elicited the Relaxation Response, makes it clear that 'just sitting quietly or, say, watching television, is not enough to produce the physiological changes. You need to use a relaxation technique [discussed later] that will break the train of everyday thought'.[20] He gives an example in his book *The Relaxation Response* of a woman with moderately high blood pressure who lowered it by regular practice of relaxation techniques.

> The Relaxation Response has contributed to many changes in my life. Not only has it made me more relaxed physically and mentally, but also it has contributed to changes in my personality and way of life . . . I feel stronger physically and mentally. I take better care of myself . . . The positive feedback which I experience as a result of the Relaxation Response and the lowered blood pressure readings make me feel I am attempting to transcend a family history replete with hypertensive heart disease . . .
>
> Intellectually and spiritually good things happen to me during the Relaxation Response. Sometimes I get insights into situations or problems which have been with me for a long time and about which I am not consciously thinking . . . I look forward to the Relaxation Response . . . I am hooked on it and love my addiction.

BIOFEEDBACK

Through the use of biofeedback monitoring, previously involuntary physiological states such as heart rate, muscle tension and skin temperature, can be brought under conscious control.[21]

The individual is connected to biofeedback instruments (by sensors attached to selected points on the body), and measurements can then be made of changes in physiological functions such as brain waves, blood pressure, heart rate or muscle tension. These changes are measured and recorded through a blinking light or beeping tone. It is possible to learn quite quickly to get the light signal or tone to alter in a desired way – by reaching a deep level of relaxation. By paying attention in this way to the feelings and sensations experienced when the signalled feedback is an indicator of relaxation or its opposite, the individual can then go on consciously to control biological functions.[22]

Biofeedback training can be used as a method for controlling adverse bodily reactions to stress, though, it must be said, not without the appropriate training and necessary equipment.[23]

Many hospitals and clinics now use biofeedback methods. Their great asset is that they lead to self-awareness. Perhaps the best results from their use have been when combined with meditation and relaxation techniques. A drawback has been that relatively expensive equipment is required for most biofeedback monitoring.[24]

Korenman, Orbach and Watson at St Bartholomew's Hospital, London[25] have recently launched 'RelaxPlus', a biofeedback system for use by health-care professionals that can demonstrate and record minute changes in an individual's relative state of relaxation.[26] This recorded state activates and changes the animation, graphs and games on screen so that the user can learn to relax and then mitigate levels of stress, improve personal effectiveness and demonstrate ability to influence health and performance.

Visualisation

Mental imagery or imaging is the technique of picturing in the mind's eye the desired changes an individual wishes to make.[27] The names of O. Carl and Stephanie Simonton, have become synonymous with visualisation, and their use of this method goes back to the early 1970s.[28]

The hypothesis for this technique is that the more clearly someone can see (picture in the mind's eye) the desired future, the more likely it is to come true. Visualisation takes advantage of what almost might be called a weakness of the body in that it cannot tell the difference between a vivid mental experience and an actual physical experience. One very important requirement for effective imaging or visualisation therefore is the development of the imagination. This is not possible for everyone (and indeed this method does not work for all), but with the motivation to succeed, coupled with help and training, it can work extremely effectively.

In his book *Love, Medicine and Miracles*,[29] Siegel demonstrates the efficacy of just such a vivid imagination in the case of a young child with a brain tumour. The child, Glenn, was taught imaging techniques at a biofeedback centre after doctors had indicated that further treatment was inadvisable. Glenn pictured the cancer as being hit by rockets and a space ship, as in a video game, and he carried this out regularly and repeatedly. After some months of so doing Glenn remarked to his father that he couldn't 'find the cancer any more', and indeed this turned out to be the case. The cancer had gone.

Researchers now believe that the images used for this technique should be ones chosen by the individuals themselves, as it is much more likely to be relevant to the individual and therefore more effective in result and should be in harmony with their own philosophy of living.

It is said to work by reducing fear and decreasing the pain which can hinder recovery. It also creates the desire for a greater degree of improvement than might have been anticipated. This in turn allows physical changes to be started as the mental processes involved influence the body's immune system. A reduction in stress ensues, perhaps allowing the possibility of the individual getting in touch with the subconscious. Finally, it allows the individual to feel that he or she is contributing to his or her own recovery.[30]

As part of a planned, structured programme to promote health-giving changes, many therapists use progressive muscle relaxation and deep breathing. Both are useful on their own, although they are often employed in combination with relaxation and visualisation with supremely effective outcomes.

Most people can learn this technique quite quickly from someone practised in the art. Some may take longer perhaps because they do not realise how easy it is to do or convince themselves that they cannot do it without really trying. Yet some people do find it difficult to visualise because they tend to think in terms of sounds or sensations rather than pictures. If this is the case, then one exercise that would help would be to sit comfortably and view a picture or a photograph for a few minutes, then with eyes closed try to re-create the scene observed in as much detail as possible.[31]

It should be remembered that creative visualisation is merely the technique of using the imagination to realise what is wanted in life and to get rid of the lack, limitation and loss brought about by thinking negatively. Some possible applications are as follows:

RELATIONSHIPS

In order to change a difficult relationship into a more harmonious one, allow yourself to relax into a quiet, meditative state. Mentally imagine the two of you relating and communicating in an honest, open and harmonious way. Experience this as if it is already happening – believe yourself that this idea is possible. Repeat this exercise often. If you are sincere in your desire and open to change you will soon find that the relationship becomes easier and the problem will be solved.[32]

HEADACHES

Allow yourself to relax deeply, close your eyes, picture a piece of pink ice in the centre of your forehead. Imagine the skin's warmth melting the ice very slowly. As this happens see and feel the resultant cool, pink liquid covering all your forehead and around your eyes. At the same time, imagine the sensation as the coolness from the melting ice penetrates your head, reducing the temperature on the inside, easing the whole of your head, the area behind your eyes and also the back of your neck.[33]

ANXIETY ATTACKS

Allow yourself to relax deeply. Close your eyes and see yourself looking at an old grandfather clock. Spend some time studying the outer casing, the hands and the numerals on the clock face and then – finally – the pendulum swinging behind the glass-fronted door. Concentrate just on that pendulum, with its slow, ponderous swing. You will find that, as you fix your full attention on the pendulum, your heart beat and your pulse rate will automatically slow to keep pace with it.[34]

CONTROL OF PAIN

Sit comfortably and relax as much as possible. Concentrate on your breathing, allowing it to become slow, gentle and rhythmic. Become aware of the pain (wherever it is in the body) and picture it as being in the shape of a circle. Direct your breathing into this circle, allowing it to become deeper, and as you do this allow the circle to become larger and larger. As the circle increases in size the pain begins to decrease. Continue until the pain has gone away. (It is natural to tense when feeling pain, so just relaxing can often get rid of it or reduce it. Using visualisation in this way is fine as long as the cause of the pain is known or being investigated.)

Uses
of relaxation

Relaxation and visualisation can be done alone or in groups, with the help of a therapist or with tapes. The best results are obtained with long-term use. Hit-and-miss efforts lead to hit-and-miss results.

In hospital settings, groups for staff and patients are useful for a regular programme of relaxation and visualisation. This can be augmented with tapes for home use.

Sessions and tapes usually begin and end with the playing of five minutes of specially composed music for relaxation, the former period to help people to break any encircling worry thoughts or to settle down after rushing to get to the group on time. The second and final phase of music allows people to go even deeper into their own levels of consciousness and perhaps experience either something of the world of the wondrous or deeper states of peace, joy and well-being. Group members and listeners are then brought back to normal awareness. It is important to be well grounded before leaving the session or room.

In groups, time should be allowed at the end of each session for comment and discussion.

The relaxation response

The basic pattern of relaxation and visualisation to obtain the Relaxation Response are as follows:

1 Sit comfortably with feet firmly fixed on the floor, spine well supported and fingers and feet uncrossed, hands lying loosely on the lap, palms facing upward. Make sure you are warm enough. Try to choose a time when you won't be interrupted.
2 Close your eyes and become aware of your breathing.
3 Breathe gently and deeply, in through the nose and out through the mouth (not longer than five minutes).
4 Allow breathing to come back to its normal level and observe its pattern, rate, rhythm and depth.
5 Tense and relax the major muscle groups of the body, beginning with the feet and finishing with the hands, noting the difference between the two.
6 Picture the colour green and feel waves of peace flowing through every part and particle of your being.
7 Sit for a while carrying out further gentle relaxing breathing. When you are ready, open your eyes.
8 You will now be able to return to your normal activities renewed and refreshed.

It is possible to relax by using only tapes. Indeed, relaxation cassettes have an important role for use at home but principally as a back-up to the work done in any group. Many people trying to carry out relaxation and visualisation techniques using cassettes alone give up sooner or later without really experiencing the long-term benefits of the techniques they are trying to do. They are then left with the idea that relaxation doesn't work. The participants in groups say that it isn't the same carrying out the exercise alone at home as doing it as part of the group. There is a feeling of safety and of being accepted in a group, and everyone benefits from this.

The following case histories show in narrative form some of the benefits of relaxation. They are included in order to show that this type of therapy can be useful to many people in many conditions. In this way the stories speak for themselves.

Case
histories

EXAMPLE OF CONJUGAL DIFFICULTIES EXPERIENCED FOLLOWING TREATMENT

Jean is a dental nurse with vast experience of working in the private sector. Although her boss, an exacting man, had a very busy practice, Jean coped with it serenely. Married to a jeweller, she has a busy social life and many interests. She has an outgoing, naturally happy personality.

And then she became ill. She developed cancer of the cervix and had various forms of treatment for it, including radiotherapy. When she resumed sexual intercourse she found to her dismay that it was painful, and this left her unhappy and demoralised, which in turn became a vicious circle as anxiety followed increasing anxiety. Her husband was totally supportive at this time and indeed throughout this traumatic period.

Her consultant referred her to the group, hoping it might help, though not perhaps really believing that it could or would. Jean was unable to attend the group sessions but regularly carried out her relaxation and visualisation exercises at home. She received detailed instructions of what, when and how to carry them out.

A close relative of Jean's is a healer, so the holistic way of life was not new to her. Nevertheless, she faithfully practised, more from a desire to find a way out of her unhappy situation than a belief in what she was doing. In any event, it was not long before there was an easing of the situation. Jean became less stressed and began to feel like her own self again.

At her next clinic appointment, three months later, Jean was delighted to be able to tell her doctor that normal relations were being resumed with relish and not pain. This consultant now regularly refers patients for relaxation.

Jean has since gone on to take up a course in stress management and now talks knowledgeably on the subject. She is very enthusiastic about the benefits of holistic medicine and in particular of relaxation and visualisation, and about how much she feels she has benefited from their use.

WIDESPREAD DISEASE

Cheryl has been struggling with cancer for five and a half years. Her first operation was for breast cancer. Four and a half years later Cheryl was told that she had developed secondaries in a hip, and a couple of months after that she had liver metastases.

And yet now Cheryl can look back at how she felt last year and say,

> How much better I feel now! I know I have changed, but am convinced that it is only with the daily 'time for myself' that I have managed to get this far. I look forward to each day as it comes now and really take pleasure in whatever it has to offer. I feel fulfilled on a personal level and am sure that my relationship with my nearest and dearest is closer than ever.

Cheryl is married with a family who were very supportive throughout her ordeal.

Relaxation seemed to help her at first in some ways, but she still worried greatly about her situation. Fears would sometimes completely overwhelm her. She then began to realise that if her worries and fears had such a powerful bearing on her disease and could actually make her feel worse, why not replace them with more encouraging, hopeful and positive thoughts with which she could actually enjoy living.

It was after this realisation that relaxation and visualisation began to help her more and more. As her attitude changed so she began to feel better. Cheryl pictured her chemotherapy working and this helped her through eight months of this treatment, which passed without any problems; indeed, her son thinks that she is now becoming addicted to the chemo, as she feels so good on it.

Cheryl's last scan, a month ago, showed another significant improvement, and because she responded so well she is to have a further two treatments. Cheryl affirms that she feels better each time she has the chemotherapy treatment. She intends keeping up the good work with the visualisation for she knows that this has been so important in helping her.

On a lighter note, Cheryl says that she is enjoying walking and cycling more than ever and in the last few months has taken up painting again, joining a class at the local adult education centre.

DEPRESSION AND SUPPORT FOR A RELATIVE

Brian, a middle-aged man, was referred for relaxation and visualisation therapy by his consultant and support team. Brian was undergoing biological therapy for a malignant melanoma. He had become very depressed, and his consultant, who really empathises with his patients, was concerned about his patient's psychological status, as he seemed so down and nothing seemed to interest him or lift his spirits.

Brian came to the group accompanied by his wife. From the very first occasion it seemed to help him. On completion of the first attempt, Brian's spirits had lifted, to the joy of his wife who said, 'You look better already!' Brian and his wife came regularly to the group and carried out the exercises at home using his relaxation tape.

After each session group members are asked to reveal what colour they chose at a particular point in the visualisation. One day Brian chose violet, for which one interpretation is creativity. Later he asked his wife to buy him some coloured felt-tipped pens, for Brian felt inspired to do some artwork. He gained the greatest amount of satisfaction and pleasure from this. One result is that the group now has a beautifully illuminated notice for its use, which is displayed on the door in order to prevent interruptions whilst a relaxation group is in session. Brian went on to produce sheets of poetry most carefully illustrated. One poem was entitled 'A Hug', extolling the benefits of the same. One line went as follows: 'No need to fret about your store of them, the more you give, the more there is of them.' This was read out to the group, who were delighted to share Brian's obvious pleasure at being able to produce such lovely artwork.

The relaxation group helped Brian's wife almost as much as it helped him as his treatment progressed. She had been through such a difficult time watching him become increasingly depressed and yet seemingly unable to help him come out of it.

WISH FOR PREGNANCY

Marney joined the relaxation group rather tentatively. She had a specific, single reason for coming. She didn't feel particularly stressed, she did not suffer from arthritis, high blood pressure or sinusitis; none of these things were relevant in her case. Her problem – if she had one at all – was that she wanted to be pregnant!

Her past medical history revealed that Marney had endometriosis. She had had a laparoscopy, and was put on appropriate medication to break up the ensuing adhesions. She herself felt that there was 'a block' preventing her pregnancy.

Some five years previously Marney and her husband decided that it was time to start a family. As the desired result did not materialise, Marney decided to take matters into her own hands. Someone, along the way, suggested relaxation and visualisation. Marney wasn't exactly carried away by the idea but she decided to give it a go anyway.

Being a member of the group proved pleasant for Marney, and she discovered the added benefits such as sharing views and meeting with people she grew to know and like.

This is a rather short story as Marney had been coming to the group only for about three months when she did indeed become pregnant. Imagine her delight at being able to share her news with the group. Marney continued to attend relaxation until going on maternity leave.

She is now back at work having had a beautiful baby boy. Life at the moment is too full to allow for relaxation classes but . . . she knows where they are and has expressed her intention to join in from time to time.

CLINICALLY WELL, EMOTIONALLY IN PIECES

Beryl, a social worker, came to the relaxation and visualisation group after becoming very aware that although she was physically fit again after having treatment for cancer for seven months, emotionally she had not dealt with the impact of the illness. She knew that this could affect her recovery. In an unpublished article she wrote to express her thoughts on the subject, she says,

> Knowledge about the physical aspects of treatment – surgery, radiotherapy, chemotherapy, etc. – is widespread and fairly freely discussed. The emotional aspects of cancer – the fear, anxiety and anger – are much less so. Yet, in any recovery from illness, the stress of the emotional impact can affect recovery. It is logical, therefore, that attention should always be given to the way a patient is reacting emotionally, and it is within this aspect of health that relaxation training can be such a support to cancer patients.
>
> When I learned I had cancer I felt overwhelmed with fear. It was the illness that I had always dreaded. I will never forget the sense of terror when I heard the news. Nevertheless, I decided to look

positively to the future and concentrate on working my way through the treatment and getting better. After seven months of treatment I constantly felt tearful, I was tense and anxious and churned up inside . . . I was introduced to the notion of relaxation training. The relaxation exercise was demonstrated to me on a one-to-one basis . . . A sheet of paper was given which clearly and explicitly explained the method – I was advised to practise at home. This I attempted to do. However, my attempt to master the technique on my own was almost a complete failure. To achieve the right pacing while remembering the instructions and to acquire the perceived benefits was just too much to attempt to do.

Despite all these thoughts, the first time I experienced the group I felt a truly wonderful sense of well-being at the end. It was the memory of that feeling which made me realise the worth of continuing with the process. As time went on, my capacity to go with the words increased, and with this, the ability to relax grew. My self-consciousness went away, and the familiarity of the routine, instead of becoming boring, somehow freed me to be taken along by the words more easily. With any learned process, the more skilled one becomes the more one gains from it, and this is true of relaxation and visualisation.

As one gains confidence in the exercise, it becomes possible to use a tape of a group in session as a valuable support at home. Relaxation and visualisation as a technique can be carried into one's everyday life and can act as a continuous support.

As to my own situation, I have a stressful job in which many demands are made on my time. When I first returned to work I experienced some loss of confidence, as is often true after a period of absence. Because of the relaxation and visualisation I found that I was more aware than I used to be of times when I was feeling tense and anxiety was building up. This awareness of my body's reaction allowed me consciously to relax and to take stock for a few minutes. In this way I overcame situations where I might have begun to feel overwhelmed by the pressure. The advantage I now find is that I am generally somewhat calmer than I was and, perhaps, a little less inclined to be short-tempered. Clearly all the pressures are still there, but the difference is that I am managing to control them and my reaction to them.

At home I use the tape of the relaxation and visualisation session. I find that, when I end a workday feeling tired and under pressure, if I then use the tape it seems to give me energy for the rest of the evening.

References

1   L. Ryman, Relaxation – supportive therapy in the treatment of cancer, Paper presented at **New Directions in Cancer Care Conference**, *Royal Marsden Hospital*, 12–13 Nov. 1990.

2   M. Snyder, Progressive relaxation as a nursing intervention: an analysis, **Advances in Nursing Science**, 6 (3): 47, Apr. 1984.

3   E. Jacobson, **You Must Relax**, 5th edn. rev. and enlarged, *London: Souvenir Press*, 1977.

4   H. Benson and M.Z. Klipper, **The Relaxation Response**, *London: Collins*, 1977.

5   Reader's Digest Association Ltd, Visualisation therapy; picturing your way to health, in **Reader's Digest Family Guide to Alternative Medicine**, *London: Reader's Digest Association Ltd*, 1991.

6   Y. Konno and K. Ohno, A Factor Analytic Study of the Acceptance of Relaxation through Dohsa Training (Psychological Rehabilitation Training) **Shinrigaku Kenkyu** [*The Japanese Journal of Psychology*], 58 (1): 57, Apr. 1987.

7   A. Meares, **Strange Places, Simple Truths**, *Glasgow: Collins*, 1979.

8   A. Meares, Stress, meditation and the regression of cancer, **Practitioner**, 226 (1371): 1607, Sept. 1982.

9   J. Chang, Using relaxation strategies in child and youth care practice, **Child and Youth Care Forum**, 20(3): 155, 1991.

10 I.S. Asaenok, L.M. Spetsian and N.A. Laysha, [Experiences in Using Rooms for Psycho-Emotional Relaxation at an Engineering Plant] **Gigiena Truda i Professionalnye Zabolevaniia**, (6): 50, June 1988.

11 Personal communication.

12 D. Goleman, Relaxation: surprising benefits detected, **New York Times**, 13 May 1986.

13 G. Stevens, Mind control, **Oracle**, 1(1): 50, Apr. 1992.

14 C. Patel, M.G. Marmot, D.J. Terry, M. Carruthers, B. Hunt, and M. Patel, Trial of relaxation in reducing coronary risk: four-year follow-up, **British Medical Journal**, 290(6475): 1103, 13 April 1985.

15 Goleman, ibid.

16 Ibid.

17 D. Mast, J. Meyers and A. Urbanski, Relaxation techniques: a self-learning module for nurses: Unit II, **Cancer Nursing** 10(4): 217, Aug. 1987.

18 Ibid.

19 Benson and Klipper, **The Relaxation Response**.

20 Ibid.

21 O.C. Simonton, S. Matthews-Simonton and J.L. Creighton, **Getting Well Again, a Step-by-Step, Self-Help Guide to Overcoming Cancer for Patients and Their Families,** *London: Bantam Books,* 1978.

22 C.L. Cooper, R.D. Cooper and L.H. Eaker, **Living with Stress,** *London: Penguin Books,* 1988.

23 Ibid.

24 L. Chaitow, **Your Complete Stress-Proofing Programme; How to Protect Yourself Against the Ill-Effects of Stress, Including Relaxation and Meditation Techniques,** *Wellingborough, Northants: Thorsons Publishers,* 1985.

25 Personal communication.

26 'RelaxPlus', Ultramind Ltd, 5 Ravenscroft Avenue, London NW11 0SA; tel. 071–982 6092; fax. 081 455 3828.

27 Simonton, Matthews-Simonton and Creighton, **Getting Well Again.**

28 Ibid.

29 B.S. Siegel, **Love, Medicine and Miracles,** *London: Rider,* 1986.

30 U. Markham, **The Elements of Visualisation,** *Longmead, Shaftesbury, Dorset: Element Books,* 1989.

31 Reader's Digest Association Ltd, **Visualisation Therapy.**

32 S. Gawain, **Creative Visualisation,** New York: Bantam Books, 1982.

33 U. Markham, **The Elements of Visualisation,** *Longmead, Shaftesbury, Dorset: Element Books,* 1989.

34 Ibid.

Further Reading

B. Roet, **All in the Mind? Think Yourself Better,** *London: Macdonald Optima,* 1987.

B.S. Siegel, **Peace, Love and Healing,** *New York: Harper & Row,* 1989.

C.M. Cade and N. Coxhead, **The Awakened Mind: Biofeedback and the Development of Higher States of Awareness,** *Longmead, Shaftesbury, Dorset: Element Books,* 1979.

D.A. Bakal, **Psychology and Medicine,** *London: Tavistock Publications,* 1979.

D. Chopra, **Quantum Healing,** *New York: Bantam Books,* 1989.

D. Zohar, **The Quantum Self,** *London: Bloomsbury,* 1990.

F. Capra, **The Turning Point,** *London: Flamingo,* 1983.

A Course in Miracles; The Text, Workbook for Students and Manual for Teachers. *London: Arkana,* 1985.

H. Selye, **The Stress of Life,** Rev. edn, *New York: McGraw-Hill,* 1976.

J. Borysenko, **Minding the Body, Mending the Mind,** *New York: Bantam Books,* 1988.

J. Madders, **Stress and Relaxation: Self-help Ways to Cope with Stress and Relieve Nervous Tension, Ulcers, Insomnia, Migraine and High Blood Pressure,** 3rd edn, *London: Macdonald Optima,* 1987.

J. Silva, and P. Miele, **The Silva Mind Control Method,** *London: Grafton Books,* 1980.

K. Walker, **The Conscious Mind,** *London: Rider,* 1962.

L.L. Hay, **You Can Heal Your Life,** *London: Eden Grove Editions,* 1987.

N. Cousins, **Anatomy of an Illness as Perceived by the Patient,** *New York: Bantam,* 1981.

N. Cousins, **Head First, Biology of Hope,** *New York: Dutton,* 1989.

G. Zukav, **The Dancing Wu Li Masters; an Overview of the New Physics,** *London: Rider,* 1979.

R. Thomson, **Loving Medicine,** *Bath: Gateway Books,* 1989.

U. Fleming, **Grasping the Nettle: A Positive Approach to Pain,** *London: Collins Fount Paperbacks,* 1990.

Cassettes Relaxation and/or Visualisation

Dick Sutphen. Probe 7 – Beyond subliminals
  1 Eliminate stress
  2 Radiant health
New World Cassettes, Paradise Farm, Westhall, Halesworth, Suffolk IP19 8RH

Louise Hay
  1 Cancer: discover your healing power
Airlift Book Co., 26 Eden Grove, London N7 8EF

Matthew Manning – self-help tapes
Matthew Manning Centre, 39 Abbeygate Street, Bury St Edmunds, Suffolk Tel. 0284–769502

BHMA (British Holistic Medical Association)
    1 Duncan Johnson, PhD. Imagery for relaxation
    2 David Peters, MB, ChB, DRCOG, MFHom, MRO. Coping with stress
    3 James Hawkins. Coping with persistent pain
BHMA, 179 Gloucester Place, London NW1 6DX
Tel. 071–262 5299

NFSH (National Federation of Spiritual Healers)
    Audrey Murr-Copland
        1 Healing light. Imagery and music
        2 The temple meditation. Imagery and music
    Jean Dreghorn
        1 Relaxation of body and mind
        2 Simply relaxing
NFSH, Old Manor Farm Studio, Church Street, Sunbury-on-Thames, Middx
TW16 6RG

Dr Chandra Patel
    1 Relaxation and meditation
4 Furze Hill, Purley, Surrey CR2 3LA
Tel. 081–660 3293

Ursula Fleming
    1 Relax to ease stress
    2 Relax to ease pain
    3 Relax to concentrate
Ursula Fleming Tapes, PO Box 1902, London NW3 2UF

Ursula Markham
    Relaxation Cassettes
The Hypnothink Foundation, PO Box 154, Cheltenham, Glos. GL53 9EG

New World Cassettes
    Dick Sutphen. RX 17
        1 Radiant health
        2 A calm and peaceful mind
        3 Creative visualisation
        4 Sleep like a baby
        5 Ultimate relaxation
New World Cassettes, Paradise Farm, Westhall, Halesworth, Suffolk IP19 8RH

New World Videos
    Dick Sutphen. Video hypnosis
        1 Ultimate relaxation
        2 Positive thinking
        3 Un-stress
New World Cassettes, Paradise Farm, Westhall, Halesworth, Suffolk IP19 8RH

Music for Relaxation

1	Legend	Peter Howell
2	Temple in the forest	David Naegele
3	Fairy ring	Mike Rowland
4	Silver wings	Mike Rowland
5	Tranquillity	David Sun
6	Harp of gold	Patricia Spero

New World Cassettes, Paradise Farm, Westhall, Halesworth, Suffolk IP19 8RH

Portraits – music for relaxation by Annie Locke, available from Mysteries, 9 Monmouth Street, London WC2 9DA

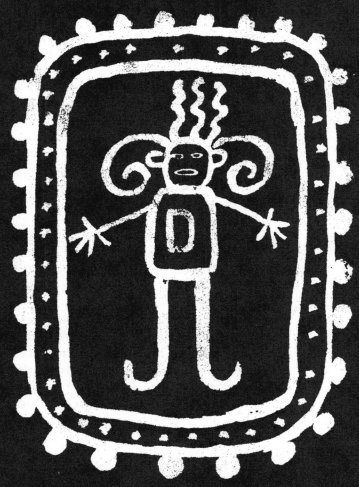

5

HYPNOTHERAPY

Sheila Conachy

The word *hypnosis* has long been synonymous with the occult and the mystical. The aim of this chapter is to demystify hypnosis and to help health professionals realise the full potential of this very powerful therapeutic tool. The history, theoretical background and principles will be outlined and discussed using case histories to demonstrate the clinical applications of hypnosis.

Hypnosis is a day-dream or trance-like state in which persons can relax, drift away and make use of the resources of the unconscious mind. It is a state of altered awareness, a profound state of relaxation, in which persons are open to suggestion. The client must *will* it to happen, *expect* it to happen and *allow* it to happen.

For many years the concept of hypnosis was discarded by the medical profession as being unscientific and smacking of quackery. As a result of much valued work and research over the past three decades, hypnosis has been given the respect it deserves in the world of the healing arts.[1]

The term *hypnosis* comes from the Greek word *hypnos*, meaning sleep. At present scientists and researchers do not fully understand the exact nature of hypnosis. Theorists state, however, that hypnosis is a state somewhere between sleep and wakefulness: an altered state of consciousness. The hypnotic state is produced by *constant repetition of a series of monotonous rhythmical sensory stimuli*, which may be visual, auditory or tactile.

Hypnosis is a natural state that can be induced by oneself or another for a specific purpose. It is a therapeutic tool, but not a therapeutic end in itself. As a method of treatment, hypnosis facilitates a number of different treatment modalities and is used in conjunction with other approaches to alter psychophysiological states, promote understanding and allow for creative problem solving.[2]

According to Erickson and Rossi, hypnosis is 'a communication of ideas and understandings to a patient in such a fashion that he will be most receptive to the presented ideas and thereby motivated to explore his own body potentials for the control of his psychological and physiological responses and behaviour'.[3]

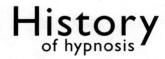

History
of hypnosis

Healing in a trance state is one of the oldest of the medical arts. The historical antecedents of hypnosis are found in the ancient writings of the Egyptians, Chinese and Indians, where the laying-on of hands, incantations, music and rhythm induced the 'temple sleep'.[4] Believers were known to have performed great feats of psychophysiological prowess, such as lying prone on a bed of nails or walking over hot coals.

In the Shang dynasty (1900 BC) dancing and singing were used to induce 'prophetic ecstasy' in individuals.[5]

In the Old Testament there are examples of the hypnotic character of several of God's activities: 'For the Lord hath poured out upon you the spirit of deep sleep, and hath closed your eyes' (Isaiah 29:10). The New Testament reveals, in the cures wrought by Jesus and the Apostles, the use of eye-fixation, the laying-on of hands and verbal suggestion: 'Jesus saith unto him, Rise, take up thy bed, and walk' (John 5:8).

The Jewish rabbis were knowledgeable in hypnotic phenomena, although many of the practices were relegated to the category of 'sorcery'.[6]

The Druids were active in hypnotic-related rituals during the first millennium AD.

In the history of hypnosis the eighteenth century is usually considered to be Mesmer's century. The word *mesmerise*, meaning to hypnotise, fascinate, spellbind, is derived from the name Mesmer. Franz Anton Mesmer (*c.* 1734–1815) is credited with being the founding father of hypnosis. He practised medicine as well as his newly labelled technique of 'animal magnetism' in Vienna. His reputation, fame and showmanship gained him not only attention and a constant flow of patients, but also a certain notoriety among his medical and academic contemporaries. Mesmer believed that disease was caused by an inharmonious distribution of magnetic fluid in the patient's body. Part of his technique was to apply artificial magnets to his patients. Diseased parts of the body were stroked with magnets, thus effecting cures, and redistributing the magnetic fluid and restoring balance within the individual. However, Mesmer soon gave up the use of magnets in preference to his own personal 'magnetism' and ability to influence the magnetic fluid of others through his own movements.[7] Mesmer did not invite scientific scrutiny of his claims and ended up professionally ostracised and isolated.

Sigmund Freud (1856–1939), the founder of modern psychoanalysis, studied hypnosis and mesmeric techniques under Charcot, in Paris, in 1885. He soon became disillusioned with hypnosis, as his patients were not always able to achieve the level of hypnosis he desired for his explorations into nervous disorders. He subsequently abandoned it as a treatment method.

In the middle of the twentieth century Milton H. Erickson became the best-known practitioner of medical hypnosis. He was born in Nevada in 1901 and died in Phoenix, Arizona, in 1980. He contracted polio as an adolescent and was able only to move his eyeballs. This enabled him to develop the art of astute observation and learn the complexities of non-verbal communication. He became aware of the importance of paying attention to inflections in the voice. Although Erickson was originally told that he would never walk again, he learned to walk by studying the progressive movements of his baby sister, who was crawling, and applied them with practised concentration.[8] His most notable professional achievements were the founding of the American Society of Clinical Hypnosis (ASCH) in 1957, and the *American Journal of Clinical Hypnosis* in 1958. Erickson used the individual's own internal processes for therapeutic intervention. He was renowned for his success with resistant clients, as he employed individualised visualisation techniques.

The American Medical Association officially accepted hypnosis in 1958, after much research, as a 'tool' to be used by the medical profession. The association strongly recommended that instruction in the use of hypnosis be included in the curricula of medical schools.[9]

Uses
of hypnotherapy

Hypnosis has been employed for various clinical and non-clinical conditions, from simple relaxation to boosting self-esteem, because of its ease of application and significant lack of side effects. There is little doubt that hypnosis can help clients with psychosomatic and other psychologically related problems.[10] Hypnotherapy, the clinical application of hypnosis, may also help clients to learn new behaviour and overcome maladaptive ones. It is now widely practised in psychotherapy, in pain clinics and in dentistry.

Hypnosis can be used as a method of anaesthesia for any surgical, obstetrical or dental procedure. It is useful in casualty departments for minor surgical and orthopaedic procedures, especially if the patient has consumed a heavy meal, which would contra-indicate the giving of a general anaesthetic. In major procedures, hypnosis has proved to be more beneficial when used as an adjunct to drugs. Hypnotic techniques used in anaesthesia produce fewer post-operative complications and promote a faster recovery.[11]

Hypnosis will be most effective in conditions accompanied by strong emotional components, such as anxiety and phobias. The greater the need for hypnotherapy felt by clients, the more readily and deeply they will respond. Hypnotherapy can be very effective in helping people to reduce weight and to give up smoking.

PAIN

Controlled experiments carried out in the research laboratories of Harvard University led to the conclusion that pathological pain is much more susceptible to suggestion than artificially induced pain. The association of anxiety with acute pain is documented in both clinical and experimental research.[12] Reduction of anxiety usually leads also to reduction of pain. The severity and prognosis of the illness or injury have profound effects on the experience of pain. Terminal illness, the loss of a limb or permanent loss of functioning will exacerbate pain perception; a transitory injury like a sprained ankle will hurt, but the pain will not be intensified by the fear and anxiety that accompany more permanent and disabling conditions.[13] Chronic pain seems to trigger psychological responses such as depression, anger and withdrawal.

The more clients feel that they can be in control of the painful situation, the higher the pain tolerance will be. Hypnosis relieves pain, reduces the anxiety and discomfort of tests and treatments, helps maintain appetite, decreases side effects from chemotherapy and radiotherapy, and promotes an active and relatively hopeful emotional state.

Hypnosis in gynaecology and obstetrics is proving to be an effective tool in allaying many anxieties and discomforts that women experience.[14]

OTHER USES OF HYPNOTHERAPY

Hypnosis and hypnotic techniques can be useful adjuncts to the medical management of hypertension and other cardiovascular problems.[15]

Hypnosis is often used effectively to help students gain more efficiency in their studies. Lack of attention, distraction and the inability to concentrate can interfere with the efficient use of the mind.[16]

Hypnosis, relaxation and visualisation all evoke an altered state of consciousness and produce a trance-like state. Hypnosis works purposefully towards creating a deeper altered state of consciousness where usual superego functions (those relating to the moral part of the personality) are temporarily suspended.

Relaxation focuses on a physiological softening of muscles; imagery utilises and depends on mental processes; each, however, may be used to promote the other.[17] Hypnosis employs both relaxation and imagery in the induction procedure, but neither is necessary for the individual to enter a trance. Yet hypnosis is more than just another form of relaxation. Although relaxation techniques are used in hypnosis, hypnotic induction does not always require relaxation.[18] Hypnotic analgesia has been found to produce more pain relief than relaxation alone.

The nature
of hypnosis

Before outlining the principles and techniques of inducing the hypnotic state it is necessary to consider the nature of hypnosis and the important parts played by the unconscious mind and the power of suggestion.

Trance is a natural phenomenon. Bored in a dull lecture, for instance, our attention wanders; we focus inwards and become absent, while still alert and awake. We go where our day-dream has taken us. Sometimes, when travelling long distances, we don't remember passing familiar landmarks, and then 'come to' with a start wondering how we got there so quickly. The trance state, a 'wakeful dissociative' state, is often synonymous with the hypnotic state. This state is recognised by a glassy-eyed stare, lack of mobility and unresponsiveness to external stimuli. A person in a trance state is more receptive to suggestion than normally.

According to Erickson and Rossi, in a therapeutic trance state, the limits 'of one's usual frame of reference and beliefs are temporarily altered so one can be receptive to other patterns of association'.[19]

Suggestion is a term used to describe an idea presented to the client for uncritical acceptance. The degree to which the client is inclined to accept uncritically certain ideas presented is known as *suggestibility*. This is enhanced by the client's motivation, expectation and trust in the therapist. Suggestibility and the hypnotic state are closely connected, and the more suggestible the client is, the more easily can hypnosis be induced and deepened. The power of suggestion is greatly enhanced when it acts upon the unconscious mind rather than the conscious, and the suggestions are acted upon much more powerfully.

Our colleagues in advertising know never to underestimate the power of suggestion, as exposure tends to influence our daily thoughts and actions, for the most part quite unconsciously (that is, subliminally). In today's society, we are constantly barraged by suggestions, on poster hoardings and television screens, in magazines and shop windows. The power of suggestion also plays a part in the practice of medicine; for example, expensive drugs prescribed by an eminent specialist may be much more effective than identical preparations prescribed by the local doctor.

The unconscious mind is the seat of all our memories, all our past experiences, and all that we have ever learnt. The unconscious mind is a much greater part of the mind, and usually we are quite unaware of its existence. The power of criticism is restricted largely to the conscious mind. When suggestions bypass the conscious mind, as they do under hypnosis, they penetrate directly to the unconscious mind.

The response to hypnosis will depend upon the extent to which the power of criticism is suppressed and the power of rejection normally exercised by the conscious mind is removed. The depth of hypnosis will be directly related to the degree of suppression attained. Light hypnosis will occur with slight suppression; deep hypnosis, or somnambulism, will occur with complete suppression.[20] The more the conscious mind is suppressed, the more the suggestibility will increase. The unconscious mind of the client is in control in hypnosis, not the conscious mind of the therapist. The words or actions of the therapist serve only as a means of arousing or stimulating within the client past learnings and understandings, some of which have been consciously or unconsciously acquired. The client will be protected by the unconscious mind. Every hypnosis is therefore basically self-hypnosis.

Hypnosis and hypnotic techniques are tools used within the larger framework of the therapeutic relationship. Success of the therapy seems to be dependent on trust, expectation, belief and the establishment of rapport.

Approximately 90 per cent of the population can be induced into the light hypnotic state, and 50 to 60 per cent can attain medium depth,[21] provided that the subject is willing and unafraid. It is generally accepted that the more intelligent, highly motivated patient who expects a positive outcome and is able to concentrate, will be very successful using hypnosis and hypnotic techniques. Also a person who is imaginative and willing to trust is usually a good subject. Analytically minded people who seek the whys and wherefores are unlikely to be easy subjects.[22] Those members of society who are trained and accustomed to accepting instructions without question, such as children, members of the armed forces, nursing and acting professions, prove usually to be excellent subjects.

Steps
in Hypnotic Technique

There are a variety of hypnotic induction, trigger and deepener techniques. The choice of any one technique depends on the client and, to some extent, the therapist. They consist of:

1 induction,
2 trigger,
3 deepener,
4 ideo-motor response,
5 therapy, and
6 termination.

1 INDUCTION

This involves making suggestions to clients that they will imagine certain things and that they will experience certain sensations or behaviours. The most commonly used induction techniques involve eye fixation accompanied by suggestions of relaxation.

2 TRIGGER

This stimulus can be of three kinds in order to get a desired response: auditory (by the use of a certain word); visual (by the movement of the therapist's hand); or tactile (by touching the client's arm). Trigger stimuli are useful and dispense with the need for repetitive complex commands. For example, the client may be told that after a count of three, the therapist will say the word *now,* and on hearing the word *now* the client will feel three times more relaxed than before.

3 DEEPENER

This is a technique for promoting or enhancing the trance state; that is, counting backwards or forwards with the suggestion that on each count the client will become more and more relaxed.

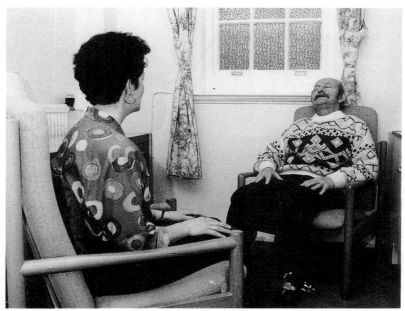

Individual hypnotherapy session

4 IDEO-MOTOR RESPONSE

IMR, or ideo-motor finger-signalling technique, is used to facilitate the client's response to questions. Once the client is in the hypnotic state, the therapist explains that a link will be established between the client's unconscious mind and, for example, the index finger of the less dominant hand. Clients can be requested to respond to questions by raising this finger, rather than responding verbally. This allows greater access to hidden subconscious material. The ideo-motor response can be of great value in communicating with unconscious patients: for example, following an accident.

5 THERAPY

Clients will have already discussed their needs with the hypnotherapist. For example, their needs might be to achieve a good night's sleep, or to be more in control of their lives and situations, or to move forward with more confidence.

6 TERMINATION

It is essential to reorientate clients back to the present time and place. This is achieved by counting back slowly – for example, from five to one – and preparing clients for reorientation back to time and surroundings.

General principles
of hypnosis

There are two types of hypnotherapy, suggestive therapy and insightful therapy. Suggestive therapy entails the therapist offering suggestions of deep relaxation. Insightful therapy includes age regression (in deep hypnosis the client can go back in time – for example, to childhood and relive experiences); dream analysis (the client is requested to dream a dream that will give insight into the problem); hypnopictography (automatic writing – during hypnosis the client draws or writes something connected to the problem); and the use of more advanced psychotherapeutic techniques.

It is normally impossible to hypnotise people against their will. In order to succeed, they must be willing and unafraid.

The most important preliminary step in the induction of hypnosis is the preparation of the client's mind. It is vital for a therapeutic outcome to spend time removing misconceptions, fears and doubts. The client's desire and willingness are evaluated and sought, and belief in hypnosis is encouraged. The symptoms are discussed and their disadvantages are highlighted. A better quality of life, without the symptoms, is emphasised. Provided that a condition is suitable for hypnotherapy, the client is told that the treatment will be effective and powerful.

Many clients are anxious and apprehensive, and will not be able to enter the hypnotic state successfully unless their fears and anxieties are allayed. People have common fears of failure, fear of domination and loss of control, fear of the hypnotic state, and over-anxiety to succeed. Most failures to induce the hypnotic state are due to inadequate preparation of the subject and inadequate discussion before induction is attempted.[23]

The *client's* will-power is the significant element in the induction of hypnosis, not the will-power of the therapist. It is always difficult (and sometimes impossible) to hypnotise very weak-willed individuals, for they cannot concentrate sufficiently to enter the hypnotic state. Conversely, strong-willed, dogmatic or self-opinionated people, provided they are willing subjects, are easy to hypnotise, because they use their will-power to force concentration. Clients are assured that they need have no fear whatever of being dominated by the hypnotherapist, and that they can never be compelled to do or say anything to which they strongly object. Even in hypnosis, people cannot be compelled to do anything to which they have rooted objections. According to Erickson and Rossi, no utilisation of hypnosis can elicit behaviour contrary to the subject's wishes, background, training, better judgment and even moral sense.[24]

Usually children are much more easily hypnotised than adults, because they are much less critical and much more amenable to persuasion and suggestion, provided that their confidence is gained and interest aroused. Children are excellent hypnotic subjects because they are natural fantasisers and have vivid imaginations.[25]

CONTRA-INDICATIONS

Proper screening of the client and the use of hypnosis by a trained therapist are essential for good practice. Hypnosis is contra-indicated in conditions such as endogenous depression, schizophrenia, psychosis and cerebral tumours. Hypnosis should be used with caution, and may be contra-indicated in people who tend habitually to retreat from reality.

The hypnotherapist uses therapeutic techniques as tools, within the therapeutic relationship, with an understanding of the client's problems and coping mechanisms. Hypnosis itself is not dangerous but can be misused if the needs of the client are not considered.

Self-hypnosis

Self-hypnosis is a self-induced hypnotic trance without the intervention of another person. In self-hypnosis, a part of the conscious mind must necessarily remain active in order to control the hypnosis and direct what is to happen in the self-induced trance. The conscious mind assumes the role of hypnotherapist in making the suggestions which enter the unconscious mind, where they are first accepted and then acted upon. Since the subject plays both an active and a passive role at one and the same time, a deep trance state is unlikely to be attained, as the subject needs to exercise conscious control.

Post-hypnotic suggestion is sometimes used to teach a subject to induce self-hypnosis. The subject who is taught in this way will be able to enter the trance much more rapidly, often in response to a self-administered signal, and will probably be able to enter a greater depth. This can be of great therapeutic value when the subject needs to induce a trance state quickly: for example, to avert an imminent attack of asthma or migraine.[26]

Subjects who have been taught to achieve self-hypnosis on their own, without the active intervention of the hypnotherapist, will always feel more in control. The increased confidence that they develop in their own unaided capacity for entering the hypnotic state when required enhances the power of their own auto-suggestions.

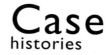

Case histories

CASE 1

Mr N was a sixty-year-old man with metastatic cancer of the bladder. He was offered a course of chemotherapy and it was explained to him that the main side effect of the regime was alopecia. The prospect of losing his hair caused him great anxiety as his body image was very important to him. Mr N chose to undergo scalp cooling in order to prevent hair loss.

The process of scalp cooling involved a heavy ice-pack being placed on top of his head for approximately one hour before every administration of chemotherapy. He soon became daunted by this procedure and would shake visibly and become very agitated. He realised that although the procedure was helping to prevent hair loss, it was also interfering with his quality of life. Mr N was given the opportunity to express his fears and anxieties, and a session of hypnotherapy was offered to him by his primary nurse. Having entered the hypnotic state, it was suggested to Mr N that every time he would feel the ice-pack on his head it would be a sign and a signal for him to allow himself to

> relax . . . deeper . . . and deeper . . . down . . . and down . . . into a deep . . . deep . . . state of physical . . . and mental . . . relaxation . . . It was also suggested that the scalp cooling and chemotherapy were working . . . with . . . him . . . and for him . . . and working with his body . . . mind . . . and spirit.

After a few sessions of hypnotherapy, Mr N's anxieties disappeared and he felt more in control and able to cope with his treatment. His wife, who understandably felt anxious and helpless, also benefited from one session. Mr N was also instructed in the art of self-hypnosis. Further questioning revealed that he suffered from claustrophobia. The cause could have been explored by using age regression in insightful therapy, but this was not considered appropriate at the time.

CASE 2

Mrs M was a fifty-four-year-old woman going to theatre for a laparotomy for obstruction. She hated the idea of having a nasogastric tube passed, and was agitated and anxious. Mrs M accepted a session of hypnotherapy when it was explained to her that the therapy would help her to relax for the procedure. After the session, she felt very calm and relaxed and easily accepted and co-operated with the insertion of the nasogastric tube.

CASE 3

K was a twenty-eight-year-old woman with abdominal metastatic cancer. She was admitted at three-weekly intervals for chemotherapy. On admission a cannula was inserted into her arm to facilitate the IV infusion of chemotherapy. K dreaded the cannula insertion, and as her condition deteriorated and her veins became more difficult to locate, so her dread worsened. It took two people to hold her arm for the cannulation as she would thrash her arms and legs around. Before every admission K became increasingly anxious in anticipation of the cannula insertion. It was explained to her that a session of hypnotherapy would help her cope with the insertion, but she declined the offer.

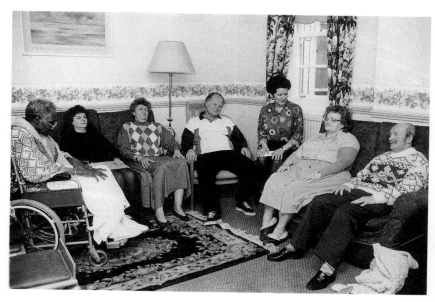

Group hypnotherapy session

Later, on hearing from fellow patients the benefits of their hypnotherapy sessions, K requested a session. K expressed her thoughts that hypnosis was synonymous with loss of control and that she feared domination. Her fears were allayed and the therapy was explained in detail. After close liaison with the IV team, K entered an hypnotic trance and was invited to allow herself to relax and use visualisation to take her to her favourite place, sitting at home, stroking her cat. Having placed a post-hypnotic suggestion that she would allow herself to enter an even deeper state of relaxation in the next session, the session was terminated.

Then, as planned, the nurse from the IV team entered the room with her trolley; K was counted back down into a deep trance and the cannula was inserted uneventfully without any discomfort to K.

Conclusion

Since the therapeutic relationship is vital to the successful use of hypnotherapy, the health-care professional is ideally placed to practise these techniques. With education and training in the art of hypnotherapy, the health professional can expand his or her repertoire and promote the quality of life of many people. Hypnotherapy is a very powerful self-help tool and an important adjunct in health care. Acknowledging the interaction of mind, body and spirit, it is also a means of facilitating the ill to help themselves.

References

1 R.P. Zahourek, **Clinical Hypnosis and Therapeutic Suggestion in Nursing**, *New York: Grune & Stratton*, 1985.

2 T. Mott, Hypnosis and phobic disorders, **Psychiatric Annals**, 11: 36–45, 1981.

3 M. Erickson and E. Rossi (eds), **Innovative Hypnotherapy – The Collected Papers of Milton H. Erickson on Hypnosis**, Vol. IV, *New York: Irvington Publications*, 1980.

4 D.C. Muthu, **A Short Account of the Antiquity of Hindu Medicine and Civilisation**, *London: Baillière, Tindall* & Cox, 1930.

5 L.B. Paton, **Spiritism and the Cult of the Dead in Antiquity**, *New York: Macmillan*, 1921.

6 S. Glaser, A note on allusions to hypnosis in the Bible and Talmud, **International Journal of Clinical and Experimental Hypnosis**, 1975.

7 W.E. Edmonston Jr, **The Induction of Hypnosis**, *New York: Wiley Interscience Publications*, 1986.

8 W.S. Kroger, **Clinical and Experimental Hypnosis**, 2nd edn, *Philadelphia: J.B. Lippincott*, 1977.

9 S. Abudarham, **Hypnotherapy in Practice**, *Birmingham: Association of Hypnotherapists in Health Care*, 1991.

10 Ibid.

11 E. Hilgard and J.R. Hilgard, **Hypnosis in the Relief of Pain**, *Los Altos, CA: William Kaufman*, 1975.

12 K.R. Pelletier, **Mind as Healer, Mind as Slayer**, *New York: Delta*, 1977.

13 P. Sacerdote, Hypnosis and terminal illness, in G.D. Burrows and L. Dennerstein (eds) **Handbook of Hypnosis and Psychosomatic Medicine**, *Amsterdam: Elsevier/North Holland*, 1980.

14 Kroger, **Clinical and Experimental Hypnosis**.

15 T.A. Wadden and C.S. de la Torre, Relaxation therapy as adjunct treatment for hypertension, **Journal of Family Practice**, 11: 901, 1980.

16 J. Hartland, **Medical and Dental Hypnosis**, *London: Baillière Tindall*, 1971.

17 R.P. Zahourek, **Clinical Hypnosis**.

18 E. Hilgard, Hypnosis in the treatment of pain, in G.D. Burrows and L. Dennerstein (eds) **Handbook of Hypnosis and Psychosomatic Medicine**, *Amsterdam: Elsevier/North Holland*, 1980.

19 M. Erickson and E.L. Rossi, **Hypnotherapy: An Exploratory Casebook**, *New York: Irvington Publication*, 1979.

20 Hartland, ibid.

21 Ibid.

22 Ibid.

23 Ibid.

24 Erickson and Rossi (eds) **Innovative Hypnotherapy**.

25 G. Garner and K. Olness, (eds), **Hypnosis and Hypnotherapy with Children,** *New York: Grune & Stratton*, 1981.

26 J. Hartland, ibid.

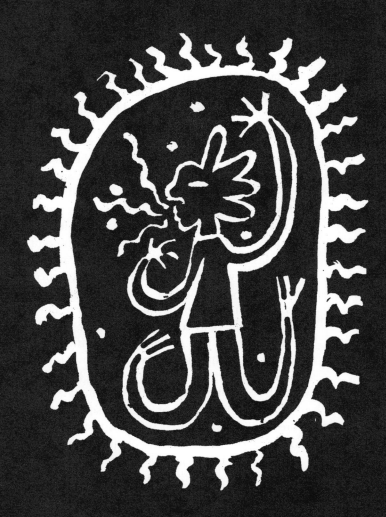

6

THERAPEUTIC MASSAGE AND AROMATHERAPY

Sheena Hildebrand

1 Therapeutic massage

Hippocrates (*c*.460–*c*.370 BC) said about a dislocated shoulder: 'It is necessary to rub the shoulder gently and smoothly with soft hands. The physician must be experienced in many things, but assuredly also in rubbing.'[1]

The word *massage* is thought to mean 'press softly' in Arabic or 'knead' in Greek. It is derived from the French word *masser*, which means to shampoo, which in turn is related to the Hindu word 'to press'.[2] This indicates how widespread the practice of massage was throughout the various civilisations. The Bible, the Qur'an and the Ayur-Veda (Art of Life) are all sacred books that mention the use of massage and aromatics to lubricate and anoint the skin.

'Massage is a systematic and scientific manipulation of body tissues performed with the hands, for therapeutic effect on the nervous, the muscular systems and on the systemic circulation'.[3] It can also be defined as a 'systematic form of touch using certain manipulations of the soft tissues of the body to promote comfort and healing'.[4] Further, massage can potentially be a powerful mode of non-verbal communication, which in a safe, therapeutic environment allows for the catharsis of emotions to occur, which may be safely dealt with by an experienced therapist.

The type of massage outlined in this chapter is aromatherapy massage. 'This is a combination of Swedish (soft tissue) massage, Shiatsu (finger-pressure) massage and neuromuscular (nerve) massage',[5] using essential oils. The oils are aromatic, volatile extracts from plants, blended into a carrier oil (a base vegetable oil). The combination of the oils and the massage allows for the senses of touch and smell to be combined for a total therapeutic effect, thus engaging as many factors together to give a truly holistic therapy, and taking into account a person's state of mind, body and spirit (see the section on aromatherapy, page 119).

Development of Massage Through the Ages

Massage is a therapy that has probably been around for as long as humanity has existed; implements for massage have been found at archaeological excavations in many countries all over the world throughout the ages.

According to research reports, in nearly all ancient cultures some form of touch or massage was practiced . . . 'These ancient civilisations used therapeutic massage not only as a pain reliever, but also to improve their sense of well-being and their physical appearance'.[6]

Ancient records from China reveal that massage was being used several thousand years ago. The technique was called 'anmo', and this spread to Japan 1,400 years ago, where it was renamed 'tuina'. It used the same principles, in that the points of stimulation to improve the circulation and the nerves were applied by a finger-pressure technique called *shiatsu* (see Chapter 7 Shiatsu).

Many other early cultures, such as those of the Egyptians, Indians and Arabs, also used massage. Western culture also included massage as a component of health care, with the practice being widely used by the Greeks and the Romans. During the Middle Ages, massage declined; however, during the Renaissance, interest in massage was renewed throughout Europe. Per Henry Ling, a Swedish professor in the early nineteenth century, formulated his own system of massage to help conditions affecting the joints and muscles. This became the basis of what is known as Swedish massage.

In more recent times several physicians – Johann Mezgar in Holland, John Grosvenor in England and Albert Hoffa in Germany – were enthusiasts in the use of massage; and it was in 1899 that Sir William Bennett inaugurated a massage department at St George's Hospital, London. There may be a number of reasons why massage did not become favoured and accepted till the end of the nineteenth century: training was of a poor standard and the women practising massage were regarded with suspicion. 'In 1894 a group of women joined together to form the 'Society of Trained Masseuses', with the intention of raising the standard and reputation of massage in this country'.[7]

In 1900 this Society became the Incorporated Society of Trained Masseuses; and in 1920 it amalgamated with the Institute of Massage and Remedial Exercise (Manchester). Subsequently, a Royal Charter was granted, and it eventually became known as the Chartered Society of Physiotherapy. State registration followed in 1964. In this century the importance of massage became even more evident during and immediately following both the world wars. This was due to the fact that during the First and Second World Wars, massage was an effective therapy for the nature of the injuries suffered. This developed into what is now physiotherapy, particularly in areas where rehabilitation was the primary treatment. As a result, massage began to have a diminished role in health care. Massage is now seeing a revival of interest, and the particular area in which it is being applied is rehabilitation. The nature of rehabilitation, however, has changed in that it is now directed towards the emotional and psychological aspects of the patients' life and well-being. The value of massage therapy is becoming more widely accepted, and its 'seedy' image is being replaced by the general public's awareness of its true therapeutic value.

In global terms, massage has evolved throughout the world in most cultures and civilisations, like any creative art form, for the purposes of enjoyment and relaxation, and as a form of therapy to help enhance the quality of life at all stages of health and illness. The challenge to health-care professionals is to integrate it safely within the present health-care setting, as a therapeutic intervention, at appropriate times in the management of a patient's condition.

The British National Health Service appears now to be taking more seriously the challenge of assimilating therapies such as massage and aromatherapy as part of patient care. This movement is particularly being initiated because of the huge interest taken by nurses in advocating improved quality of life, and improved standards of care for patients and their families. The potential for massage to enhance a patient's quality of life in many health-care settings is apparent: for example, in care of the elderly, neonatal care, midwifery, care of the dying and in oncology.[8–12] Many nurses are taking up the challenge to train in the therapy, and following it by appropriate integration of the use of touch therapy (which maybe a form of simple touch, massage, shiatsu, reflexology or aromatherapy) as part of the development of their communication skills.

Therapists are also beginning to address the issue of evaluating the effects of such therapies. For example, a study of the effects of aromatherapy in the intensive care unit has recently been undertaken at Battle Hospital, Reading, which will be available shortly,[13] as has another study at the Middlesex Hospital, London.[14] There is clearly a need for scientifically validated research in this field and there is much that is currently in progress.

The Royal Marsden Hospitals in London and Surrey offer therapeutic massage with essential oils as part of their holistic approach to cancer care, and will be conducting a study.[15] This will examine the effects of massage (with essential oils) on cancer patients' perceptions of their quality of life, symptom distress, and levels of anxiety and depression. The study will use a three-group (a control group, a group receiving massage, a group receiving massage with essential oils), pre- and post-experimental research design.

The British Medical Association's Report on Alternative Therapy suggests that time, touch and compassion are three elements that are not exclusive to the alternative therapist, but which a medical practitioner may sometimes not apply because of pressures or lack of time and resources, and this may in fact play a crucial part in the belief of the therapy by the patient. Their view of aromatherapy is described thus:

> The way a therapist uses the touch of hands on a patient can reinforce a sick person's confidence, and reinforce the will to recover full health. A particular example of the use of deliberate techniques of this kind is given by aromatherapy, which seems almost entirely to be based on the caring, reassuring and pleasing effects of touch.[16]

The Marylebone Health Centre was one of the first GP practices in London to employ a massage therapist. The service is given as part of the conventional treatment available for the patients. The Marylebone Centre Trust, which is affiliated to this health centre, run massage training courses for nurses, doctors and other interested health-care professionals.

The International Therapy Examination Council (ITEC) is a body which sets standards that can be considered as a way of obtaining a recognised qualification, but there is at present no one universal standard accepted by all the various schools, and the various professions interested in integrating the therapy in their curriculum.

Effects of Massage

Massage can affect the patient in a number of ways.

Physically, massage can affect most of the body's systems[17] to:

1 help eliminate metabolic wastes;
2 decrease blood pressure;
3 increase circulation of the lymph fluid, thus helping to drain nodes that may be sluggish;
4 relax or stimulate muscles;
5 relieve tension, stiffness and aches in muscles and joints;
6 help respiratory muscles to relax and to aid deep breathing;
7 improve tone, elasticity and circulation to skin;
8 relieve restlessness and insomnia, promote a sense of well-being and help relieve pain.

Emotionally, massage can create a therapeutic 'space', relieving stress and allowing catharsis to occur. (These effects will be outlined in greater detail in the next section of this chapter.)

Massage Movements Based upon Swedish Massage Techniques

TOUCHING

This can be superficial or deep, and involves the therapist in applying touch to the client without movement in any direction. It 'attunes and focuses' the therapist and the client together to achieve a calm, relaxed state within both the client and the therapist.

EFFLEURAGE (STROKING)

This can also be superficial or deep, and involves moving the hands over a part of the client's body with varying degrees of pressure. Superficial stroking is always used on the return of the movement away from the heart and deep stroking is used when working towards the heart in order to aid circulation.

PETRISSAGE

This involves kneading with the fingers and thumb of each hand in a circular direction. It is a vigorous movement with the purpose of stimulating the muscles and assisting venous and lymphatic flow.

FRICTION

This involves movements such as wringing, rolling, compression, circular friction, and transverse friction, all of which enable deeper muscle penetration to take place. Also joints are worked around by using the palm or heel of the hand, or thumbs, or fingers.

TAPOTEMENT (PERCUSSION)

This involves movements such as tapping, slapping, and beating, which are quick vigorous, rhythmic movements to stimulate and tone muscles.

VIBRATION

This involves a continuous shaking, trembling movement either from the therapist's hand or from an electrical appliance to a specific part of the client's body. This can bring about relaxation and release of tension if applied lightly but can have a numbing effect if left for too long.

Shiatsu Massage

Shi- means finger and *Atsu* means pressure in Japanese. This massage works on the principles of Ki and yin-yang. Ki is the life force or energy which is considered to be the substance which underlies mental, emotional and physical health.

Yin-yang are considered the polarities of Ki, and represent the elements of the feminine and masculine principles in each of us. Yin can be defined as passive (or negative) and yang as active (or positive). Shiatsu involves applying finger or thumb (or even the palm or heel of the hand, or elbow) pressure along the energy flow of the meridians, which are invisible lines with points that are thought to connect with the organs of the body. As they complement each other, they are known as either yin or yang meridians. Yang meridians all flow down the body from head to foot, and yin meridians all flow up the body from feet to head. An assessment can be made to identify if a client is more yin or yang, and pressure along meridians is applied accordingly. We are constantly a mixture of both yin and yang, although sometimes one or the other may be dominant (see Chapter 7 Shiatsu).

Neuromuscular Massage

This method has been developed by western osteopaths and masseurs. It is a form of deep massage which is intended to reach nerves, ligaments, tendons and other connective tissue not normally reached by soft tissue, performed with the pads of the thumbs and/or fingers.[18]

Manual Lymph Massage

This is a gentle technique which involves stimulating the lymphatic system to help drain the lymphatic fluid, and to encourage the removal of waste products. This is performed by using gentle, circular strokes in an upward direction to the proximal lymph nodes, working out towards the extremities. This technique is becoming very popular, and is particularly useful in helping patients with lymphoedema problems; for example, a patient with breast cancer who has lymphoedema in her arm following mastectomy, or a man who has advanced prostate cancer and has lymphoedema in his legs. However, the therapist needs to be well practised, have medical consent, and use the massage in conjunction with other methods to help lymphoedema.

Aromatherapy Massage

This involves the use of a combination of the following movements with a blend of essential oils in a carrier oil.

1 touching (see Figure 6.1).
2 effleurage/stroking (see Figures 6.2, 6.3 and 6.4).
3 Shiatsu – the deep thumb pressure can be varied: with no movement, with pressure by small circular movements, or by sliding the thumb along the meridians.

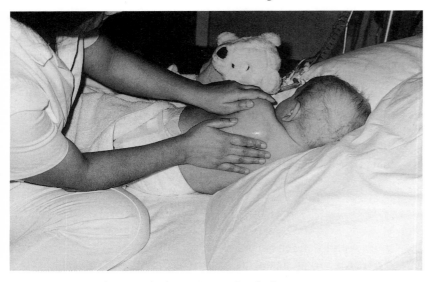

Figure 6.1   Touching: at the beginning and end of massage

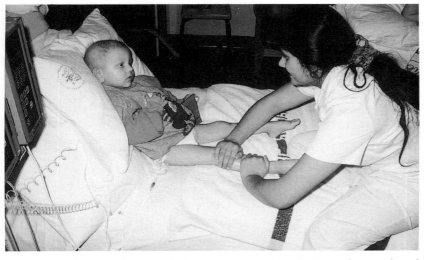

Figure 6.2   Effleuraging the whole leg to improve circulation and strengthen the muscles at the beginning of massage

The aim of aromatherapy massage is to help the penetration of the essential oils into the body, to aid relaxation or stimulation, to treat specific areas of the body, and to treat the whole body via the nerve supply, reflexes and the meridians.[19] For this to occur the massage has to flow, with the movements blending into each other so as not to break contact. The therapist has to work, with physical concentration on the movements, and to feel calm, confident and relaxed. This is to ensure that the clients feel totally relaxed and able to let go of their own tension. If the therapist feels tense, upset or negative, this will inevitably be reflected in the results of the massage, as so much is communicated with the touch of the therapist's hands. Massage is a wonderful therapy in that it is not only enjoyable to receive, mesmeric and hypnotic to watch, but also relaxing to give. It is unique in that it can be learned at any age and be enjoyed by everyone at any age. This is because the basis of massage is touch, and touch is instinctive – for example, rubbing an elbow, or massaging the temples to relieve a headache. Touch is a very important form of communication in any health-care setting. Of the five senses, touch is the most 'sensitive', but one that is sometimes the least attended to, particularly in the clinical situation, where touch tends to be for technical and mechanical purposes (such as in the intensive care unit). This also explains the current interest within the nursing profession to explore ways to improve direct patient contact for a more healing, meaningful and positive purpose.

It can be observed that the Western approach to massage is to demonstrate that the therapy is based upon definite scientific principles, but the Eastern approach is much more subtle. It is based upon opening invisible channels of energies, looking at the person as an organism interacting within itself, with others, and the universe itself, thus giving it a holistic rather than a technical meaning.

In order for a therapeutic experience to occur, the following are necessary. Firstly, *communication skills*: the most important factors in creating a therapeutic environment are for the therapist to have an empathetic approach, an open mind and a non-judgemental attitude towards the client. An approach such as this will allow for safe emotional release that may occur as a result of the hands-on treatment. To achieve this the therapist needs to have his or her own sense of self awareness, and to be experienced in communication and counselling skills.

Secondly, *knowledge*: to ensure safety in a health-care setting the therapist should be appropriately

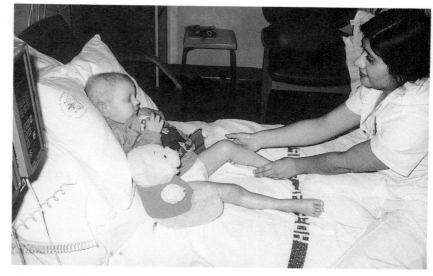

Figure 6.3 Effleuraging the calf near the end of the massage

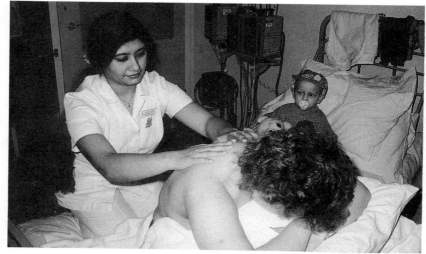

Figure 6.4 Effleuraging the patient's mother's back for relaxation

trained in the use of therapeutic touch, massage and of essential oils. In addition, the therapist should have a thorough knowledge of anatomy and physiology as it is essential to know how the human body functions. In a specific health-care setting it is also necessary for the professional therapist to have knowledge of different illnesses, the treatments involved, the effects of the treatments, and their prognosis. This not only gives understanding of the physical and psychological effects of a disease process, but also allows the therapist to assess when massage can be of benefit, and when it may be contra-indicated.

Thirdly, *environment*: in creating a pleasant physical environment the therapist will aid the process of relaxation. A warm, quiet room is essential, with suitable dim lighting and the means to warm the towels. A range of music which is relaxing can add to the experience. The décor of the room should be soft, with warm colours that are not distracting to the eye. However, if none of these facilities is available, this does not mean that therapeutic massage cannot take place, as the most important factor is the intention to give a nurturing, compassionate, sensitive touch therapy for the purpose of relaxation, healing and relief of symptoms.

Benefits

'The mind, which before massage is in a perturbed, restless, vacillating and even despondent state, becomes after massage, calm, quiet, peaceful and subdued; in fact, the wearied and worried mind has been converted into a mind, restful, placid and refreshed,' wrote the Victorian doctor Stetch Dowse in 1887.[20]

Case Histories

The cases below focus on patients suffering from various types of cancer, but the potential of the use of therapeutic massage can be easily transferred to any health-care setting.

CASE 1

A forty-year-old woman with cancer of unknown origin, and widespread bone metastases, was admitted for pain control, and for staging of her disease. She was referred for therapeutic massage because of her understandably high levels of anxiety and back pain. On her first admission she was given a half-hour massage with a blend of lavender (*Lavandula officinalis*) and rose otto (*Rosa centofolia, R. damascena*), essential oils in grape-seed oil (base/carrier oil). This is how she described the experience:

> I felt very relaxed once the treatment had started. It seemed to relieve every ache and pain in my body. The massage was very soothing and seemed to relax the tightness in my neck and shoulders. In a word, 'Heaven'.

Only the lightest of touch and superficial effleurage strokes were used repeatedly to obtain this effect.

CASE 2

A woman in her early sixties with breast cancer who had had breast surgery several days before was referred because of tension and aches and pains in her neck. She had a very light back massage with lavender (*Lavandula officinalis*) and bergamot (*Citrus bergamia*), essential oils blended in grape-seed oil. This is how she described the effects of the massage:

> I consider the massage treatment I had today has been very beneficial in relieving the muscle tension and post-operative pain associated with my breast operation. I would recommend that this treatment be offered to other patients in similar circumstances.

CASE 3

A fifty-year-old woman with advanced breast cancer was referred for relaxation because of her high levels of anxiety. She was given massage to both legs and feet with a blend of neroli (*Citrus aurantium amara*), lemon (*C. limon*) and bergamot (*C. bergamia*), essential oils in grape-seed oil. She had three sessions over a week, during which she was able to express her fears, anxieties and sadness at her situation. She was able to cry during the sessions and expressed feeling better for having shared her feelings. This is how she described her experience:

> Therapeutic massage is wonderful. It makes me feel very tranquil and relaxed. As I lie there a sense of peace comes over me. I can't recall feeling that tranquil anywhere else. After the massage my legs have a lovely pulsing feeling. She seems to draw the tension out of me while doing the massage. I lie there and I am at peace with the

world. It is a lovely feeling. I hope others can benefit from it as much as I do.

CASE 4

A forty-three-year-old man admitted with a carcinoma of unknown origin with bone and lung metastases was referred on the patient's own request because of aches and pains and to aid relaxation. He was seen five times before he died. Usually he would want his back, legs or feet massaged. He very much liked the blend of lavender (*Lavandula officinalis*), sandalwood (*Santalum album*) and bergamot (*Citrus bergamia*), essential oils in grape-seed oil. This is how he described his experience:

> Soft, awakening, smooth, totally painless massage. Continuation of movement provides excellent soothing effect and both physical and indirectly mental relaxation. It can be considered as the brightest spot in a patient's day in hospital.

CASE 5

A woman in her fifties diagnosed as having an insulinoma with liver metastases was referred for relaxation. She had a rare disease with a poor prognosis. She was seen three times before she was transferred to a hospice, where she died. This is how she described the therapy:

> I found the process of gentle movements in therapeutic massage to be relaxing, and the use of the oils enhanced the procedure. For the remainder of the day I was more alert, and the itching in my legs from fluid retention was greatly reduced. I appreciate the service being offered in the hospital and hope that it is just the beginning.

CASE 6

A forty-eight-year-old man was admitted with a T-cell lymphoma. He was referred to therapy because of aches and pains all over his body but particularly his legs. He was seen four times, and his wife was taught how to massage him as she was very keen to learn how to help her husband in any way possible. She was able to learn the basic principles of light, gentle massage, and describes how they both felt about the therapy:

X finds the treatment helps him to relax. His skin condition has improved; it was very dry around the feet and legs. His words when asked how he felt about the treatment: 'Fantastic'. For myself I have enjoyed seeing X relax and I feel I've learnt a lot so that I can continue to help X. At the same time I feel more relaxed, which is good for both of us.

CASE 7

A forty-seven-year-old woman diagnosed with carcinoma of the anal canal, admitted for investigations into undiagnosed pain in the groin area, was referred for relaxation, and because of the pain she was experiencing. She was seen regularly and was helped to relax. Her pain was persistent, and she was eventually diagnosed as having a recurrence of the tumour. However, she always said that the therapy at least made her symptoms bearable. This is how she describes her experience:

'Quiet, restful, peaceful and calm'–words such as these only just begin to describe the loving touch, the healing touch and inner healing from spirit and mind that I experience when I have a session. My mind floats away quietly in complete relaxation.

These are just a handful of comments written by patients who feel they have benefited from therapeutic massage. A content analysis of the written comments identified the following perceptions for patients who received the therapy: relaxing and soothing, reduces pain, sense of well-being and healing, peaceful and tranquil, reduces tension, and stimulating and beneficial. Other effects noticed by patients include improvement in skin conditions, relief from itchiness, help in sleeping, and help with dyspnoea.[21] Since the main reasons for referral were for relaxation, stress, depression, tension and anxiety, aches and pains, dyspnoea and insomnia, and nausea and vomiting, the results appear to justify the use of aromatherapy in this health-care setting.

The other main benefits, which should not be underestimated, are the fact that time is spent on a one-to-one basis, for at least half an hour to an hour, sometimes more, which is usually uninterrupted. However, the above experiences are anecdotal in nature, and there is a clear need for further specific investigations into the actual benefits of massage and essential oils.

Sims in her paper 'Slow stroke back massage for cancer patients' gave this summary:

The results of a pilot study undertaken to examine the effects of gentle back massage on the perceived well-being of six female patients receiving radiotherapy for breast cancer are described. An experimental approach was taken, with pre- and post-measures of symptom distress and mood, using the subjects themselves as their own controls. The patients reported less symptom distress, higher degrees of tranquillity and vitality, and less tension and tiredness following the back massage, when compared with the control intervention. The small scale of the study and the lack of statistically significant results limit the extent to which the findings can be generalised. They suggest, however, that gentle back massage may be beneficial for certain patients and that further research is warranted in this area.[22]

Another study, by McCorkle, investigated the effects of touch as non-verbal communication on sixty seriously ill patients between the ages of twenty and sixty-four, hospitalised on general medical and surgical units in the University of Iowa Hospitals and Clinics, Iowa City, assigned to experimental and control groups (thirty each).

Results of this study demonstrated that the nurse can establish a rapport with a seriously ill patient within a short period of time. The findings support the use of touch for indicating to seriously ill patients that the nurse cares about the patient.[23]

The benefits of therapeutic massage in pain relief have also been related. Pain is defined as being 'whatever the experiencing person says it is, existing whenever he says it does',[24] 'Pain is influenced by expectations, past experiences, suggestions, anxiety, depression, and other psychological factors', and as 'anxiety increases pain intensity, decreasing anxiety leads to decreases in pain perception',[25] so potentially therapeutic massage can be used as a tool to aid communication, reduce anxiety, increase comfort and thus reduce perception of pain.

Applications of Therapeutic Massage

It must be stressed that when working in a health-care setting that the professional and accountable therapist is working with the consent of the medical team involved with the patient, and also with the patient's consent, or that of the next of kin if the patient is unable to give consent for any reason.

Precautions and Contra-indications

There are precautions and contra-indications that the therapist must take into account:

1 Ensure that the patient understands the purpose of therapeutic massage, as any misunderstandings over the intent of touch can lead to embarrassment on both the therapist's account as well as that of the patient.
2 Avoid massage in infectious or contagious skin conditions or disease, as this may spread the infection from one area of the body to another, as well as to the therapist and/or to any one else the therapist treats.
3 Avoid massage during pyrexia as this may increase the body's temperature further.
4 Avoid massage over recent scar tissue or open wounds.
5 Avoid massage where the patient has a deep vein thrombosis, as there is a possibility of a clot breaking off and producing a pulmonary embolus.
6 Avoid massage in acute, undiagnosed back pain, especially if sciatica occurs as massage may exacerbate the pain.
7 Avoid massage over undiagnosed pain and inflammation.
8 Avoid massage over fractures and bone metastases.

This is not a complete list of do's and don'ts, but brief guidelines for safe practice. When dealing with patients with cancer it is advisable to do the following:

1 Use a very light, gentle, superficial effleurage technique, using soft, slow, soothing strokes. This allows for complete relaxation to occur.
2 A whole-body massage can be extremely draining and tiring even for the healthiest of people. It is best to choose a part of the body that the patient feels he or she may enjoy and also an area that is distal to the pathology; for example, a patient with a brain tumour may find massage to the legs and feet very relaxing. Often the relaxing effects of concentrating on one area permeates throughout the body, particularly if working on the feet. This may be explained by the fact that massaging the feet can be extremely relaxing, but also because reflex points on the feet are being pressed (see Chapter 9 Reflex Zone Therapy).
3 Avoid massage directly over the tumour and affected lymph nodes.
4 Avoid massage over radiotherapy areas until at least ten days after radiotherapy has finished, and consult the radiotherapist first.
5 If a patient is having chemotherapy or hormone therapy, it is best to

assess the individual as to whether it is suitable to give therapeutic massage. Patients may feel too ill during the chemotherapy to want a massage, even if it is very gentle, especially if they have never experienced it before. If they have benefited from the therapy before, it may help them to cope with the side effects of the treatment.

6   If a patient has a low platelet count (thrombocytopenia), then extreme care has to be taken as massage may cause bruising. If the count is extremely low, then massage should be avoided altogether, and instead use simple touch techniques to aid relaxation.

7   Lymphoedema: see manual lymph massage (page 109).

8   Most treatments in oncology can cause skin to be hypersensitive to touch and irritation. It is wise to adjust the massage technique and dilution of essential oils, so that only touch that is painless and enjoyable is used, and that the aroma of the oils is light and subtle.

These are only guidelines, and it is up to the therapist or health-care professional to assess individually if a patient may benefit from therapeutic massage at a particular time during treatment.

Summary

Therapeutic massage can be defined as manipulation of the body tissues performed by the hands for effect upon the nervous and muscular systems, and on the systemic circulation.[26] It can also be considered as a very powerful mode of communication from one human being to another, by using the sense of touch, especially in the health-care setting where sometimes it may be the only way to communicate positively with an individual one cares about. The use of essential oils profoundly enhances the experience of massage, although this needs to be further validated by scientific research.

The benefits of massage have also been illustrated by the case studies, particularly the psychological benefits of creating a trusting, therapeutic relationship, which allows for a truly holistic experience to occur. This is vitally important when dealing with vulnerable, disabled patients in any health-care setting. It is also important to work alongside the medical team involved with the patient, to have their consent and the patient's consent before treatment, taking into account when it is beneficial to massage and when it is not.

It is clear from the case studies included in this chapter that massage provides a number of therapeutic benefits. It is encouraging to see that a number of studies exploring the therapeutic benefits of massage have been completed, and others are proposed.

Therapeutic benefits can be demonstrated by the application of scientific approaches, which should include self report techniques and quality of life measures. However, a subjective experience of a therapy that is tailored to an individual's needs – in particular, to emotional and spiritual needs – will remain unable to be measured if it is only looked at clinically and with so-called 'scientific' principles.

Massage is a very positive, universal method of showing other human beings that they are cared for; used appropriately in health-care settings, massage can improve the quality of life and well-being of patients and their families.

'Love is the pursuit of the whole' – *Plato*.

II Aromatherapy

Look in the perfumes of flowers and of nature for peace of mind and joy of life.

Wang Wei, 8th century AD

Aromatherapy is a treatment using essential oils of plants (non-oily aromatic extracts of plants) in a controlled way to achieve balance and harmony in the human mind, body and spirit. Each essential oil possesses therapeutic qualities from the plant from which it has been extracted, and has its own particular 'aroma' or fragrance.

A treatment of aromatherapy should involve a full consultation with the client, allowing a total assessment to be made of the client's health and health concerns. A professional aromatherapist will then be able to choose a blend of essential oils dissolved in a suitable vegetable carrier oil for a body massage that will be individually tailored for that client to meet his or her individual needs for that day. This should be followed by general advice on the use of essential oils for the maintenance of good health and for dealing with stress. As aromatherapy involves the 'hands-on treatment', using the sense of touch and the sense of smell in the inhalation of the oils, combined with creating a therapeutic environment to allow for a therapeutic effect or healing to occur, it can be considered as one of the most holistic and enjoyable therapies one can experience. However, aromatherapy is not simply a massage with aromatic oils, as the essential oils can be administered and used in other ways (see below).

The use of aromatic essences and what are known as essential oils goes back to far ancient times in the same way as do the history and use of massage in ancient civilisations. The purpose of their use was often for the treatment of illness and for religious rituals. The Egyptians used the oils for embalming the dead, to beautify themselves and as offerings to their gods. Several oils are mentioned in the Bible: frankincense, myrrh and hyssop. They were known in China in the earliest of times, and in Britain as well, through the assimilation of Greek and Roman culture.

Hippocrates, a great advocate of massage and the essences, said: 'The way to health is to have an aromatic bath and scented massage everyday'.[27] However it was only when Avicenna, the great Arab physician, developed the distillation process in AD 1000, that essential oils as they are now known, were effectively extracted. In the Middle Ages, interest grew in the use of plants and herbs for healing and warding off plague and illnesses. But by the late nineteenth century chemists had begun to learn and categorise the chemical components of essential oils and to isolate what was considered to be therapeutically useful and then synthetically produce substances that were cheaper. Aromatherapists, however, believe that as a whole the chemical components of essential oils have a balancing effect on each other and that by removing part of the essential oil its synergistic effect is lost.

In the early twentieth century, a French chemist, René-Maurice Gattefosse, is credited with coining the term 'Aromathérapie' after his research on the use of essential oils in dermatology. Jean Valnet, a surgeon in France, used essential oils in the treatment of wounds during the First World War, and his book, translated as *The Practice of Aromatherapy*, is still an important textbook for professional aromatherapists today (see Further Reading). It was an Austrian woman, Marguerite Maury, a surgical assistant and nurse with a keen interest in botany and biochemistry, who developed the technique of blending the essential oils for use in application with massage. Although initially used in beauty therapy, aromatherapy is now being recognised for its full therapeutic value and is growing to be one of the most popular therapies in the health-care setting.

What are Essential Oils?

'An essential oil is a fragrant, volatile liquid extracted by distillation from a single botanical source.'[28] These oils can be extracted from various parts of plants, such as the flowers, seeds, leaves, fruits, bark and roots. The chemical constituents of each individual essential oil can be very complex, and most of the components are in the chemical families of the alcohols, ketones, aldehydes, terpenes, phenols, esters and several others. All essential oils are volatile but they have different rates of evaporation. They are inflammable, so should be kept away from direct flame or heat. It is best to store the essential oils in the dark, in amber bottles and away from extremes of temperatures. Essential oils are soluble in vegetable oil, fat and alcohol but only slightly soluble in water. Essential oils have a life of 18 to 24 months, and it is best to discard any after this length of time.

The purity of an essential oil depends on the process of extraction (which can be distillation, expression, maceration, cold process 'enfleurage' or solvent extraction process), the quality of the plant, the soil it is in, the season, and even the time of day it is picked, and most importantly, the honesty and integrity of the supplier. The cost of a pure essential oil depends on the amount secreted by the various parts of the plants. A poor yield will mean that the oil will be expensive and not easily available – for example rose otto (*Rosa centifolia, R. damascena*) – and a good yield will mean that the oil will be cheaper and more easily available – such as eucalyptus (*Eucalyptus globulus*).

How do Essential Oils Work?

It is not known exactly how essential oils work, but it is believed that they can penetrate the skin (blended in vegetable carrier oil as in the application with massage) through the pores and hair follicles, reaching the blood capillaries, thus entering the bloodstream and then reaching other bodily systems. The other main method is through inhalation, when the essential oil particles affect the olfactory system via the nose, eventually affecting the area of the brain associated with smell, triggering various neurochemicals which may be sedative, relaxing, stimulating or euphoric in effect.[29] Essential oils can be ingested too, but most professional aromatherapists tend to achieve the effects of the essential oils on the mind through the sense of smell; to apply them by the massage technique; and to cause inhalation into the lungs through the nose. However, what makes an aromatherapy treatment have a profound effect, particularly on the emotional and psychological state of a person, is difficult to analyse. It seems to be a combination of the actual physiological and psychological effects of the oils chosen, the therapist's touch and massage technique (this may be intuitive and a combination of Eastern and Western techniques), and a created therapeutic 'space' allowing patients to express themselves in a safe and trusting environment. Also, an experienced professional aromatherapist may use other principles to enhance the treatment and make it a more holistic experience, such as using crystal therapy, reflex points on feet and other approaches.

WHAT ARE CARRIER OILS?

Carrier oils are vegetable oils used in aromatherapy massage to carry out massage movements evenly over the body area and, most importantly, to help the essential oils to penetrate the skin. A good carrier oil is 100 per cent pure refined oil, cold-pressed, and it should have no aroma of its own. Examples of good carrier oils are grape-seed, olive, sweet almond and peach-nut. Wheat-germ and avocado oils are good for dry skins, but too rich, heavy and expensive to be used on their own.

How to Use Essential Oils in a Health Care Setting

1 *Inlation* A few drops (4–8) of essential oils (a combination of 2–3) are put on a paper tissue which can be placed between the pillow and pillow-slip, or drops on a piece of cotton wool can be pinned to clothes. This method is particularly useful when a decongestant is required – e.g., eucalyptus (*Eucalyptus globulus*), lemon (*Citrus limon*), pine (*Pinus sylvestris*) – as well as being an effective way to help with anxiety and insomnia with essential oils such as lavender (*Lavandula officinalis*), benzoin (*Styrax benzoin*) and bergamot (*Citrus bergamia*).

 This is a very simple and effective way of administering aromatherapy in a ward setting, especially on night duty, as the aroma tends to permeate the patient's own bed area but not necessarily disturb anyone else should they not like the aroma.

2 *Bath* 5–10 drops are added to a bath prepared to a comfortable temperature. The patient soaks in the bath for a minimum of ten minutes. This method allows the oils to work both directly by absorption of the oils through the skin and by inhalation of the aromatic vapours. It is of benefit for general aches and pains, or anxiety before an operation, and can induce a feeling of well-being

with essential oils such as lavender (*Lavandula officinalis*), chamomile (*Anthemis nobilis*), rosemary (*Rosmarinus officinalis*) or juniper (*Juniperus communis*).

3 *Foot and hand baths* 4–5 drops are placed in a bowl of warm water. Steep hands or feet for at least 10 minutes. This method can be used effectively to relieve the pain of arthritis and reduce inflammation with essential oils such as chamomile (*Anthemis nobilis*), or lavender (*Lavandula officinalis*) or juniper (*Juniperus communis*).

4 *Massage* 1–3 drops in 5 ml of carrier oil or lotion should be massaged over the desired area. The therapeutic benefits of massage have already been discussed, and the oils used for this method should be chosen to treat the patient's total needs and accord with the patient's preference.

5 *Room freshener* 10–12 drops in a small bowl of warm to hot water are set near a warm place (e.g., near a radiator or a suitable burner that does not infringe health and safety rules). This method can help to mask unpleasant odours caused by infected wounds or incontinence, as well as deodorising the clinical area with pleasant and fresh smells. Suitable oils are mandarin (*Citrus reticulata*), lemon (*C. limon*), and rosemary (*Rosmarinus officinalis*).

These are just a few ways in which aromatherapy could be used in the ward setting, and would enhance the quality of life of a patient in any setting if implemented with care and innovation.

PRECAUTIONS

There are a few important points that must be considered when using the essential oils:

1 If a patient has a history of being allergic to several substances, then it is advisable to do a 'patch' test before a full treatment is given – e.g., before massaging a patient with a blend of essential oils in a vegetable carrier oil. Apply the mix to a small area with the essential oils and to another area without the essential oils and leave for several hours. If there is no reaction, then carry on with the treatment. Always watch for any reactions such as irritation and inflammation.

2 Never use essential oils neat on the skin, and avoid direct contact with mucous membranes, in particular the eyes.

3 If the patient does not like the aroma of the oils, then it is best to start again, mixing a blend the patient likes, as there will be little psychological benefit if the patient finds the aroma offensive.

4 Increase the dilution of the essential oils if the patient's sense of smell is altered due to treatment or illness, as in the case of cancer patients undergoing certain regimens of chemotherapy. The use of essential oils may not be appropriate at that particular time.

5 In pregnancy (whether that of the therapist or the client), essential oils need to be carefully chosen and used. A professional aromatherapist should have the required knowledge to do so.

An experienced therapist should be able to judge the appropriateness of the various methods of therapy and tailor them individually to the patient's needs in collaboration with the health-care team concerned with the patient.

Case Histories

Here are two examples of patients given aromatherapy massage for whom the smell of the essential oils had quite an effect.

CASE 1

L was a young woman who had been battling with her non-Hodgkin's lymphoma for many years and her disease was progressing fast. She referred herself for aromatherapy to help her relax and to ease her increasing pain, loss of appetite and nausea. She had several sessions, all of which enabled her to relax, ease her pain and also helped her reduced appetite. This is how she described the effects of the essential oils: 'The smell of the oils is enough to make me feel high! A very clear, light, and refreshing smell, pleasing to the nose.' This was after the use of neroli (*Citrus aurantium amara*).

In another session geranium (*Pelargonium graveolens*), rose otto (*Rosa centifolia, R. damascena*), and lemon (*C. limon*) were used. 'A slightly stronger and heavy perfume. With a feel of leafy green roses around me and the sweet smell of Turkish delight, as if waiting to be eaten in front of me.' The final session before L was discharged home for a while, she described thus:

'Such a deep relaxation of peace and contentment came over me today. Am very conscious of the breathing in of the oils which cover me all over. My breathing was very slow, deep and relaxed. My pulse and heartbeat not so quick and racy, more like the ticking of the clock, slowly winding down. The mixture of these oils are lovely. The smell of fresh lemons in the air, and yet the orange blossom (also known as neroli) just to sweeten. The bergamot, a little like the orange, but just heavier. Appetite: excellent. No sickness. Frame of mind: Good, Great, Strong, Positive'.

CASE 2

D was a woman in her late fifties with a tumour of the lungs that had metastasised so that she suffered from spinal cord compression which made her paralysed from the waist down. She had limited feeling in her legs because of this. She was referred for relaxation and because she was feeling very anxious. Lavender (*Lavandula officinalis*) and bergamot (*Citrus bergamia*) were blended with grape-seed carrier oil. This is how she described her sessions: 'Today's treatment to my legs brought warmth and a little sensation, but because of the numbness of both legs the feeling is limited, but the aroma of the oils used are once again so relaxing'.

One of the principal methods of the use of aromatherapy is with therapeutic massage, which, combined, give a holistic approach to the care of the client. Aromatherapy is not by any means fully understood, but its profound and sometimes dramatic effect on the senses has been observed through its history and was described by Mme Maury, the pioneer in aromatherapy, as 'the purest form of living energy that we can transfer to man'.[30]

Summary

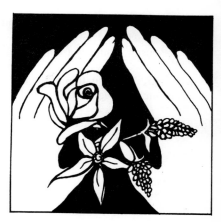

'Touch-by-Scent'

References

1   S. Price, **Practical Aromatherapy: How to Use Essential Oils to Restore Vitality**, 2nd edn, *Wellingborough: Thorsons*, 1987.

2   M. Beck, **The Theory and Practice of Therapeutic Massage**, *New York: Milady Publishing Co.*, 1988.

3   **Encyclopaedia Britannica**, Micropaedia, Vol 1, Massage, 15th edn, London: 1984.

4   E. Feltham, **Therapeutic touch and massage**, *Nursing Standard*, 5(2): 26–28, 1991.

5   R. Tisserand, **The Art of Aromatherapy**, 10th impression, *Essex: C.W. Daniel Co. Ltd*, 1990.

6   Beck, ibid.

7   A.G. Goldberg, **Body Massage for the Beauty Therapist**, 2nd edn, *Oxford: Heinemann Professional Publishing Ltd*, 1989.

8   H. Passant, **A renaissance in nursing**, *Nursing*, 4(25): 12–13, 1991.

9   L. Paterson, **Baby massage in the neonatal unit**, *Nursing*, 4(23): 19–21, 1990.

10 M. Evans, **Reflex Zone Therapy for mothers**, *Nursing Times*, 86: 29–31, 1990.

11 R. Byass, **Soothing body and soul**, *Nursing Times*, 84(24): 39–41, 1988.

12 P. Turton, **Touch me feel me heal me**, *Nursing Times*, 85(10): 42–4, 1989.

13 C. Dunn, Senior Nurse, Battle Hospital, Reading, personal communication.

14 C. Stevenson, Senior Ward Sister, Middlesex Hospital, London, personal communication.

15 J. Corner, **An Evaluation of the use of massage and massage with essential oils on the well-being of cancer patients**, *Academic Nursing Unit, Royal Marsden Hospital, London*, personal communication.

16 BMA, **Alternative Therapy**, *Report of the Board of Science and Education, London*: p. 75, 1986.

17 Beck, ibid.

18 Tisserand, ibid.

19 Ibid.

20 C. Maxwell-Hudson, **The Complete Book of Massage**, *London: Dorling Kindersley Publishers Ltd*, 1988.

21 S. Hildebrand, **Massage with essential oils – a quality of life strategy**, *Journal of Clinical Nursing*, 1(3): 114–15, 1992.

22 S. Sims, **Slow stroke back massage for cancer patients**, *Nursing Times*, 82(13): 47–50, 1986.

23 R. McCorkle, **Effects of touch on seriously ill patients**, *Nursing Research*, 23 (2): 125–31, 1974.

24 M. McCaffrey, **Nursing Management of the Patient with Pain**, *Philadelphia: J.B. Lippincott*, 1979.

25 K.M. Doehring, **Relieving pain through touch**, *Advancing Clinical Care*, Sept./Oct., 4(5): 32–3 (10 ref), 1989.

26 **Encyclopaedia Britannica**, Micropaedia, Massage.

27 Maxwell-Hudson, ibid.

28 R. Tisserand, **The Essential Oil Safety Data Manual**, *Hove: The Tisserand Aromatherapy Institute*, 1985.

29 S. Price, **Aromatherapy for Common Ailments**, *London: Gaia Books Ltd*, 1991.

30 D. Ryman, **Using Essential Oils for Health and Beauty**, *London: Century Hutchinson Ltd*, 1986.

Further Reading

MASSAGE

F. Armstrong, Scenting relief, **Nursing Times**, 87(10): 52–4, 1991.

P.E. Clark and M.J. Clark, **Therapeutic touch: is there a scientific basis for the practice?** *Nursing Research*, 33(1): 37–41, 1984.

N. Cohen, **Massage is the message**, *Nursing Times*, 83(19): 19–20, 1987.

D. Crowther, **Complementary therapy in practice**, *Nursing Standard*, 5(23): 25–7, 1991.

P. Fromant, **Let me rub it better**, *Nursing*, 4(46): 18–19, 1991.

K. Grainger, **The alternative approach**, *Nursing*, 4(46): 9–11, 1991.

A. Harrison, **Getting the massage**, *Nursing Times*, 86: 34–5, 1986.

M. Hodkinson, **Lymphoedema: applying physiology to treatment**, *European Journal of Cancer Care*, 1(2): 19–23, 1992.

C. Horrigan, **Complementing cancer care**, *The International Journal of Aromatherapy* 3(4): 15–19, 1991.

G. Joachin, **Step-by-step massage techniques**, *The Canadian Nurse*, 4: 32–5, 1983.

D. Kreiger, **Therapeutic Touch: How to Use your Hands to Help or Heal**, *Philadelphia: Prentice-Hall*, 1979.

A. Le May, **The human connection**, *Nursing Times*, 28–32, 19 Nov. 1986.

L. Lidell, **The Book of Massage: The Complete Step-by-Step Guide to Eastern and Western Techniques**, *London: Gaia Books Ltd*, 1984.

B. Olson, **Effects of massage for prevention of pressure ulcers**, *Decubitus*, 2(4): 32–7, 1989.

G.L. Randolph, **Therapeutic and physical touch: physiological response to stressful stimuli**, *Nursing Research*, 33 (1): 33–36, 1984.

P. Turton, **Joining forces**, *Nursing Times*, 31–2, 19 Nov. 1986.

J. Trevelyan, **Relaxing with massage**, *Nursing Times*, 85(3): 52–3, 1989.

J.A. White, **Touching with intent: therapeutic massage**, *Holistic Nursing Practice*, 2(3): 63–7, May, 1988.

R. Wise, **Flower power**, *Nursing Times*, 85(22): 45–7, 1989.

G. Wyatt and S. Dimmer, **The balancing touch**, *Nursing Times*, 84(21): 40–2, 1988.

AROMATHERAPY

M. Arcier, **Aromatherapy**, *London: Hamlyn Publishing Group Ltd*, 1991.

P. Davis, **Aromatherapy an A–Z**, *Saffron Walden: The C.W. Daniel Co. Ltd*, 1988.

G. Martin, **Alternative Health: Aromatherapy**, *London: Macdonald & Co. Ltd*, 1989.

M. Maury, **The Secret of Life and Youth**, *Saffron Walden: C.W. Daniel Co. Ltd*, 1989.

S. Price, **Practical Aromatherapy**, 2nd edn. *Wellingborough: Thorsons Publishers Ltd*, 1987.

R. Tisserand, **Aromatherapy for Everyone**, *Harmondworth: Penguin*, 1988.

R. Tisserand, **The Art of Aromatherapy**, *Saffron Walden: C.W. Daniel Co. Ltd*, 1977.

J. Valnet, **The Practice Of Aromatherapy**, *Saffron Walden: C.W. Daniel Co. Ltd*, 1980.

S. van Toller and S. Dodd, **Perfumery: The Psychology and Biology of Fragrance**, *London: Chapman & Hall*, 1988.

V.A. Worwood, **The Fragrant Pharmacy**, *Basingstoke: Macmillan*, 1990.

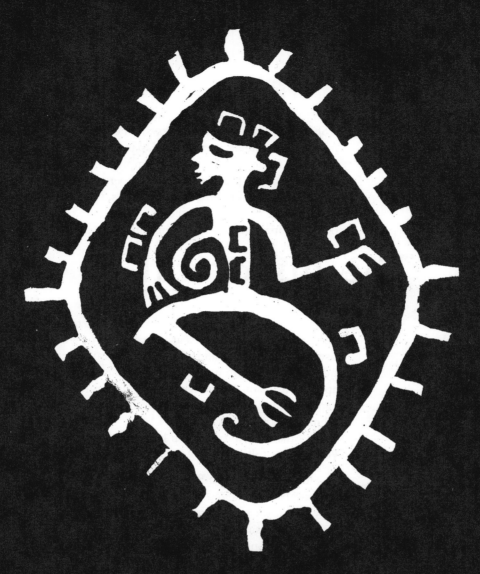

7

SHIATSU

Chris Jarmey with Verena Tschudin

Definition

Shiatsu is a physical therapy system of oriental origin. The word *Shiatsu* means finger pressure in Japanese. However, this translation is somewhat misleading, as it might imply a system where the fingers alone are used to apply pressure to another person's body. In reality, Shiatsu includes the use of palms, thumbs, knees, forearms, elbows and feet. Also, because it is given on the floor or in a chair rather than on a couch, Shiatsu emphasises maximum use of gravity to deliver its effects.

The historical
context

The origins of Shiatsu lie firmly within the roots of traditional Oriental medicine, which is at least 3,000 years old. In particular, it is based on traditional Chinese physical therapy methods known as *anmo* and *tuina*. Shiatsu in its present form emerged in early twentieth-century Japan, as a fusion of *anmo* massage, classical Oriental medical theory as used in acupuncture, plus some specific Western manipulation techniques.

The official definition given by the Japanese Ministry of Health and Welfare is as follows:

> Shiatsu therapy is a form of manipulation administered by the thumbs, fingers and palms (. . . plus elbows, knees, and feet) without the use of any instrument, mechanical or otherwise, to apply pressure to the human skin, to correct internal malfunctioning, promote and maintain health and treat specific diseases.[1]

It is only since the 1970s that Shiatsu has been widely known in Europe and the United States.

The philosophical
context

The purpose of Shiatsu is to stimulate and activate the body's self-healing and self-regulating abilities. To understand how it aims to fulfil this purpose, we must comprehend the following concepts. They are also described in more detail in the chapter on Acupuncture, where they are based on the traditional Chinese medicine. Shiatsu, coming from Japan, uses slightly different names and different spellings.

Chapters 7 and 8 treat similar subjects. Readers may wish to compare the text and tables where appropriate.

KI

The concept of *Ki* (Chinese *Qi* or *Ch'i*) is basically the same as that of modern physics, which views everything in nature as a manifestation of energy. Blood and body fluids are seen as more material forms of *Ki*, whereas thoughts are considered *Ki* in its most subtle and insubstantial form. However, in a medical context, the word *Ki* is reserved for that power which energises physiological functions and all movement. Therefore the ability to move around is directly related to the quantity and free circulation of *Ki* within the body. Likewise, the pumping action of the heart and movement of blood is also dependent upon *Ki*. Lethargy, dullness and a general lack of strength in the immune system indicates insufficient *Ki*, whereas vitality and resistance to disease reflects a high level of *Ki*.

KI CHANNELS

A system of interconnecting Channels (sometimes called meridians) links all functions and organs of the body. Part of each *Ki* Channel flows inside the body to connect with the organs, and partly near the surface of the body. Shiatsu is thus able to keep the *Ki* flowing without restriction, by way of hands-on techniques applied directly to the Channel sections near the body surface.

TSUBO

There are certain points along the *Ki* Channels where the bodily functions can be strongly influenced by pressure, as in Shiatsu, or needles, as in acupuncture. These points are known as *Tsubo*. They are surface reflections of fluctuating functional imbalances. Thus, energy can be tonified if weak, moved and dispersed if blocked, and calmed if over-active. The method of touch throughout a Shiatsu treatment will vary according to the nature of the patient's problem.

Many *Tsubo* and all the *Ki* Channels have correspondences to the mind and emotions as well as physical correspondences within the body. Consequently, Shiatsu has applications in the balancing of emotional states as well as treating purely physical problems.

YIN–YANG

In Oriental medicine, the concept of harmony and balance is expressed through the idea of *Yin* and *Yang*. *Yin–Yang* is basically the two complementary yet opposite sides of everything in the universe. As such, everything in nature has both *Yin* and *Yang* qualities – nothing is totally one or the other. The Chinese symbol for *Yin–Yang*, illustrated below, clearly illustrates that *Yin* and *Yang* interpenetrate each other and contain the seed of each other.

Yin is associated with such qualities as cold, darkness, rest and passivity. *Yang* is associated with warmth, brightness, activity and movement. Table 7.1 shows many comparisons between *Yin* and *Yang*.

This information helps the Shiatsu practitioner to formulate a treatment strategy aimed at balancing out such discrepancies in *Yin–Yang* ratios. The Shiatsu method of minimising *Yin–Yang* discrepancies, such as too much *Yang* predominating (causing restlessness, dryness and so on) is essentially the smoothing or strengthening of *Ki* flow within the Channels, mainly by stimulating specific pressure points which have documented effects upon the body's *Yin–Yang* ratio.

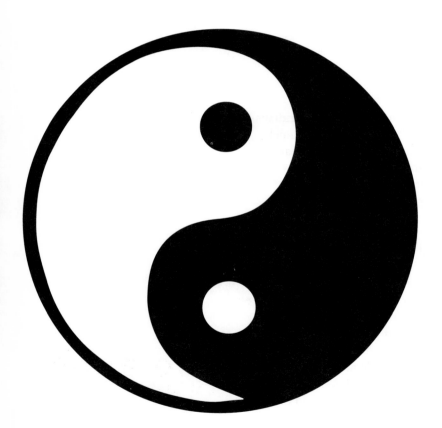

The Chinese symbol for Yin–Yang

EXCESSIVE OR DEFICIENT KI IN THE CHANNELS AND TSUBO

Any Channel or *Tsubo* may err towards lack or excess of *Ki* in relation to any other. The pattern is constantly fluctuating. The aim of Shiatsu is to discover the root cause behind any acute or chronic disharmony and attempt to stabilise it. This is achieved by tonification of deficient areas of *Ki* or dispersal of excessive areas of *Ki* within the channels.

The over-full or blocked-up *Tsubo* are easy to find because they feel 'active' and often painful, near the surface. The *Tsubo* lacking in *Ki* are more difficult to find because they exhibit little or no reaction, and are

Table 7.1 Comparisons between *Yin* and *Yang* (see also Table 8.2 on page 165)

YIN	YANG
General correspondence	
Shade	Brightness
Female	Male
Moon	Sun
Rest	Activity
Material	Immaterial
Contraction	Expansion
Soft	Hard
Within the body	
Front	Back
Organ's substance	Energy supplying organs
Interior organs	Exterior tissues – skin, muscles
Blood, body fluids	Ki
Moist	Dry
Slow	Rapid
Cold	Hot
Sinking	Rising
Clinical manifestations	
Chronic disease	Acute disease
Gradual onset	Rapid onset
Pale face	Red face
Not thirsty	Thirsty
Loose stools	Constipation
Cold	Heat
Sleepiness	Restlessness, insomnia

more hidden below the surface. By balancing these two off against each other, all the other imbalances in all the other Channels will tend to balance themselves out.

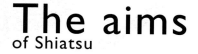

The aims
of Shiatsu

The basic aims of Shiatsu for use among family and friends and simple practice for patients are as follows:

- to help the recipient to relax, and therefore to provide a means to combat the effects of stress;
- to improve the recipient's lymphatic flow, blood circulation and vitality, and therefore to boost the immune system;

- to help alleviate aches, pains and stiffness;
- to help both the giver and the receiver to become more aware of their bodies;
- to develop healing compassion through appropriate physical contact.

The qualities
needed to give Shiatsu

The aims of Shiatsu can only be realised after certain qualities have been developed in the giver. These can be described as:

- the ability to remain relaxed and comfortable irrespective of which technique is employed at any given time;
- the ability to detect subtle changes in a person's vitality through the medium of touch;
- the ability to assess a person's level of health or disease through the development of greater empathy and the understanding of the principles of Oriental medicine.

These qualities are further highlighted in the description of Shiatsu's basic principles, as given below.

Basic principles
of Shiatsu

MOTIVATION

As with many of the complementary therapies, both recipient and giver benefit because they are in such close contact. Using one's own energy in the service of others enhances the common and universal Ki, which then floods back, to be used again. For this reason the practitioner's motivation has to be genuine. The personal qualities needed to practise are therefore also basic to the technique.

STEADINESS OF BREATH

Relaxed breathing produces an evenness of mind and body. Steadiness of breath produces a centredness in the person out of which it is possible to feel the barely perceptible changes in muscle tone, circulation and energy levels. It also leads to the sensitivity necessary to tune into the recipient's frame of mind.

CENTREDNESS

Centredness can be achieved in many ways. Most spiritual disciplines can help, particularly if they emphasise drawing the mind to the belly. The centre of the body is considered to be the lower abdomen, and its energetic centre and physical pivot point is known as the Tanden, located about 1 cm below the umbilicus. A person who is centred is someone well grounded, focused on what she or he is doing, and using the maximum potential of the body and mind together. It is essential that all movements and techniques in Shiatsu originate from the belly in order to ensure a low centre of gravity. This will make certain that one's body weight is employed rather than physical strength.

RELAXATION AND COMFORT

Good Shiatsu can relax someone, whatever the situation and circumstances. The ideal surroundings for practice are a comfortably warm room, amenable environment, and both giver and receiver clad in one layer of loose cotton clothing. Shiatsu is usually given on the floor, with a thin mat to lie on if necessary. It can also be given to a patient in bed, although this makes it more difficult for the therapist to keep a low centre of gravity, causing it to be harder work.

EMPTY MIND

Shiatsu is more about feeling than thinking; in other words, being centred in the 'gut', rather than the head. Thinking is a valid and necessary process in a Shiatsu health assessment, but basic Shiatsu is the natural act of touching and holding another human being, and as such pre-empts thinking.

SUPPORT RATHER THAN FORCE

The whole purpose of Shiatsu is to encourage the free flow of energy throughout the body and mind. To support the recipient at different levels is therefore vital. The first level of support is the fact that the recipient is going to be assisted, not imposed upon. The second level of support is to ensure stability. This involves helping the recipient to be comfortable on the floor, either prone or supine, sitting or lying on the side. The third level of support, then, is the supportive touch. If the movements are *leaning* rather than pushing, initiated from the belly, the practitioner's hand will be welcomed. The fourth level of support is to be accessible if the receiver needs to clarify any after-effects arising out of a Shiatsu session, and a word of encouragement may prove to be a highly supportive part of the treatment.

POSITIVE CONNECTION

It is impossible to support people without being connected to them. A connection can be positive or negative. In giving Shiatsu there is the possibility to make a positive connection. Connection has both a physical and psychological aspect, and an open and friendly contact will help it to be positive.

The actual pressure applied will also contribute to the positive connection. With few exceptions, having both hands in contact with the person, but kept slightly apart, works best. The giver should then focus the mind on the lower belly rather than on hands or thumbs. This will result in the receiver experiencing the two contact places as if they were one large, single area of contact. The giver will experience this as a distinct current of energy or 'echo' between the two hands. This may feel like a circle of continuity through and with the receiver, between the hands and through the belly.

PERPENDICULAR PRESSURE

Since Shiatsu is concerned with harmonising *Ki,* it is important that pressure, whether applied with fingers, palms, thumbs or knees, is applied at right angles to the surface of the body. This is because the surface distortion caused by non-perpendicular pressure tends to compress and stretch the tissues unevenly around the point of contact. Perpendicular pressure produces a centring quality by creating a steady, even epicentre of contact, which has a magnetic attraction to *Ki,* and is therefore very tonifying for that area if held for several seconds. Perpendicular pressure is even more crucial when connecting directly with a *Tsubo.* A *Tsubo* is shaped like a vase, and non-perpendicular contact will fail to get beyond its neck, and therefore make little or no contact with the Channel's *Ki.*

STATIONARY PRESSURE

The deepest Shiatsu treatment is the tonification of the deficit of the *Tsubo* most lacking in *Ki.* Stationary pressure will therefore be used more frequently than variable pressure technique. Stationary pressure is deeply penetrating and therefore able to connect with deficient *Ki,* which lies more deeply below the surface than excess *Ki.* Two to 10 seconds of pressure is generally enough, but up to 45 seconds is sometimes required.

TECHNICAL ABILITY

The skill of a practitioner is not in how many techniques she or he is able to apply, but in the proficiency in delivering them. A few fundamental techniques are all that is required. Experience will present more advanced variations. Quality rather than quantity of techniques is the key.

CONTINUITY

To receive good Shiatsu is to experience a feeling of integration throughout the body and between the body and the mind. This means that each technique should be a logical extension of the previous one, and wherever possible, contact should be maintained as the hand moves from one area to the next.

CHANNEL CONTINUITY

Shiatsu uses the fixed *Tsubo* (see the figure on page 138 and also the figures on pages 168–70) and also some transient or temporary *Tsubo* which appear spontaneously at other points along a Channel. It is therefore possible to work along an entire Channel rather than on just the classical *Tsubo* alone. By keeping a support hand stationary, and the other hand working along the course of a Channel, it is possible to feel the points which react to touch, either directly in the moving hand, indirectly in the support hand or in both. By feeling reactions between both the support and the moving hand it is possible to experience the energetic quality of the Channel, thus enabling the practitioner to follow its course via the *Tsubo* which appear within it, tonifying, dispersing or calming them as required. This is known as 'Channel continuity'.

FLUENCY

Fluency means being well practised in a wide variety of techniques. It means being able to give a full body Shiatsu, or a specific treatment without having to think about the actual technique. Fluency is only achieved with practice. It is best to practise some set techniques so that the need to decide what to do next is eliminated.

EMPATHY

Empathy is the ability to understand another person's feelings and to communicate these to him or her. A genuine concern for the other's well-being will enhance empathy considerably. When head (mind), heart

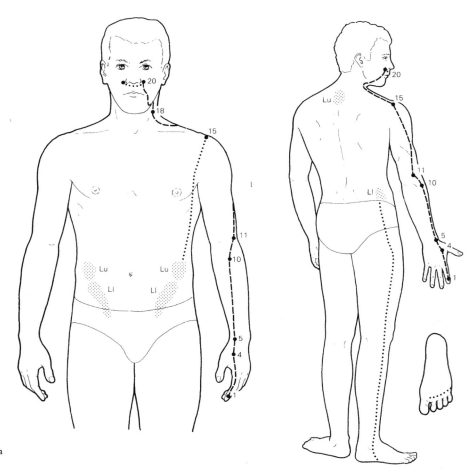

Lu = Lung diagnostic area
Li = Large Intestine diagnostic area

The Large Intestine Channel – an example of one of the 14 major Channels used in Shiatsu

and belly are open, the *Ki* is able to flow between them and between the two people, and then the conditions for giving and receiving Shiatsu are favourable.

Applying
Shiatsu

The three main ways of influencing *Ki* are by tonifying, dispersing or calming.

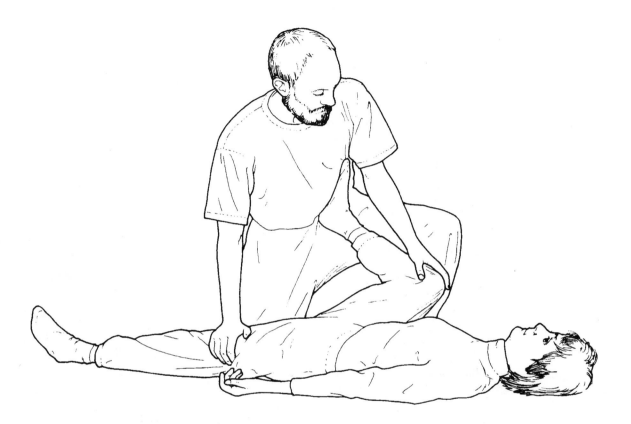

TONIFYING

In order to tonify *Ki*, stationary pressure should be applied to the mouth of a *Tsubo* with a thumb or fingertip, so that a deep connection can be made. The pressure should be held until some reaction is felt. Sometimes this feels as if the vase-shaped *Tsubo* is filling up with *Ki*. This should take from about 10 seconds to 2 minutes. If nothing is felt after 2 minutes, it is better to move to another *Tsubo*, perhaps returning later to the ones which are slow to react.

It is important that the pressure is not too deep, as this could have

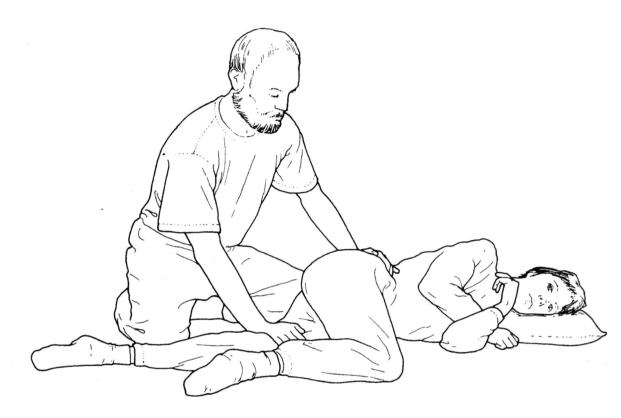

the counter-productive effect of dispersing *Ki*, as well as feeling invasive and painful to the recipient. The *Tsubo* should be approached with the attitude of meeting the *Ki*. *Ki* goes where the mind is focused. By visualising the area lying slightly deeper than a finger's depth, it is possible to be more effective with less pressure. In this way, the recipient's *Ki* will be drawn to meet the giver's *Ki*, which will then be projected slightly ahead of the fingertip. If and when a connection is felt, the pressure should be slighly reduced to allow *Ki* to fill the *Tsubo*. Broad tonification of an area can also be achieved with palms, elbows, knees or feet.

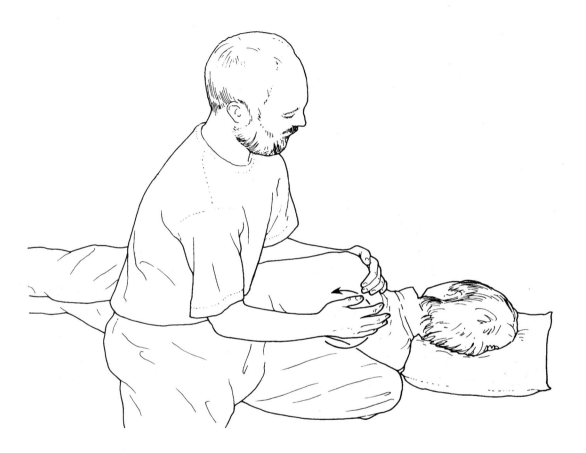

DISPERSING

The reason for using a dispersal technique is to unblock a concentration of *Ki* so that it can move smoothly along the Channel. This can be achieved by easing a thumb or finger a little way into the Tsubo and applying a rotary movement, imagining the *Ki* being loosened and dispersed. The pressure should then be progressively eased, spiralling out of the point. Alternatively, 'pumping' in and out of a slightly blocked *Tsubo* is sometimes effective. Stretching, squeezing and shaking techniques all disperse areas which are generally congested.

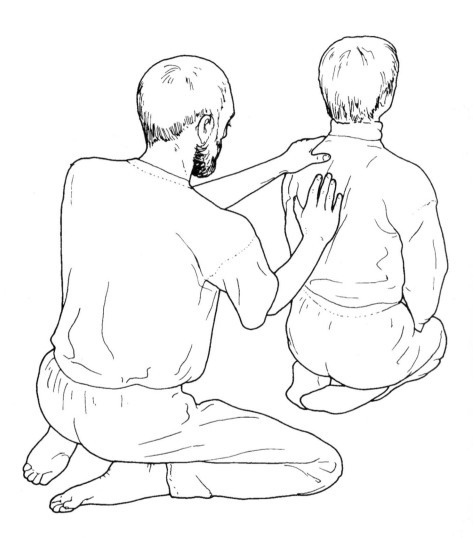

CALMING

Calming is a gentler type of dispersal. Sometimes an area of the body, or a *Tsubo*, presents a frenetic quality because the *Ki* in that area is hyperactive rather than too concentrated. In this situation, a calming technique is indicated. Calming is achieved by simply covering the area with the palms and remaining calm and peaceful.

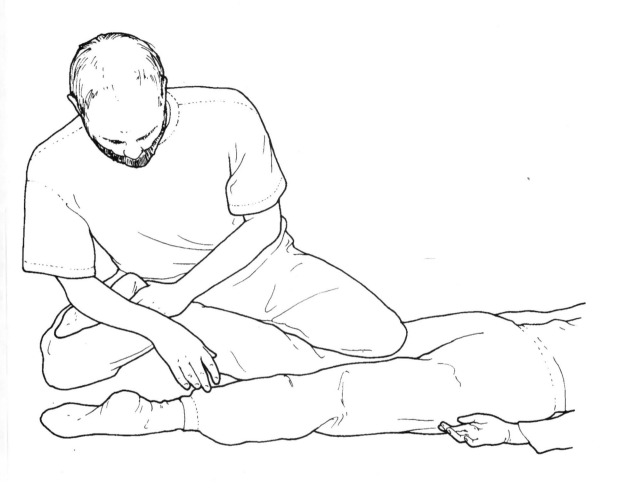

The Five Elements
in Oriental medicine

Some of the terminology of Shiatsu may be confusing to someone familiar with Western medicine. It may therefore be helpful to have some understanding of Oriental medicine, particularly its philosophical basis. The Oriental concepts of the Elements is one way to gain access to that philosophy.

In contrast to the Western four elements (earth, water, air, fire), the Orient has five Elements, which are water, wood, fire, earth and metal. Esoteric philosophers have understood the number five to symbolise dynamic interchange, and thus to represent nature. This is how the Five

Elements are best understood: as stages of transformation which interconnect on every level of the natural world, including the human being's own microcosm. Each of the Elements also relates to the various Shiatsu *Ki* Channels. The Five Elements serve the Shiatsu practitioner in three interconnected ways: they can enhance accurate physical diagnosis; provide a comprehensive model for understanding and treating the patient on an emotional level; and deepen philosophical insight.

Each Element is also linked with an attitude. Fear is linked with water, anger with wood, joy with fire, pensiveness with earth, and grief with metal. If a person is stuck in one or other of these attitudes, these can intensify into passions and so dominate the psyche. The figure below demonstrates how each of the Elements also controls one other in an effort to balance *Ki*, and *Yin–Yang*.

As an example, it can be seen that water controls fire. If the water Element becomes afflicted, both physically and psychologically, through over-work and mental strain, the kidneys (water) will fail to provide a secure foundation for the heart (fire). This allows the mind to become over-excited and nervous. When coupled with a vague sense of fear precipitated by a weakened water Element, feelings of anxiety may result.

Understanding the cause of anxiety from this perspective allows Shiatsu practitioners to formulate an appropriate and effective treatment strategy. In this particular case, they should consider tonifying the Channels and associated areas of the kidneys as well as dispersing those of the heart. Particular emphasis could be given to treating specific *Tsubo* which strengthen the *Ki* of the kidneys, and calm the mind.

The Five Elements are therefore of practical value in Shiatsu. They can, at the same time, be of spiritual value to the healers. As a dynamic model of wholeness they can allow them to look at their own lives and assess, in a non-judgemental way, the relative balance of the different

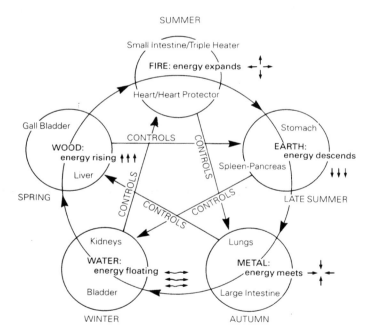

The Five Elements

parts in their own lives. How do they touch their own deepest core and renew themselves (water)? Is there a harmonious sense of achievement in their lives, being neither driven nor without vision (wood)? Can they allow themselves to love and so be essentially self-fulfilled (fire)? Do they truly listen to life, integrate experience and allow it to change them (earth)? Do they feel connected to others, neither cut off nor impinged upon (metal)?

The concept
of physiological function in Oriental medicine

Most Channels are named after an organ. However, as already mentioned, the oriental medical view of each organ is wider in connotation than in Western medicine.

These functions should not be equated with the Western concept of organ function; that would only lead to confusion. To distinguish them here, when using the Oriental concept, a capital letter is used.

The twelve Organs are classified in pairs. Each pair contains one Organ which is more *Yin* and one which is more *Yang*. Thus we have six pairs of Organs.

Yin **Organ**	*Yang* **Organ**
Kidneys	Bladder
Liver	Gall Bladder
Heart	Small Intestine
Heart Protector	Triple Heater
Spleen	Stomach
Lungs	Large Intestine

THE KIDNEYS

The Kidneys' main function is to store concentrated *Ki* known as 'Essence', which governs birth, growth and reproduction. In particular, the Essence controls bones, teeth, the brain, the spinal cord and nerves. The Essence also enables the ears to function, and the hair to remain healthy and abundant.

Because the Kidney Essence is necessary for reproduction, the Kidneys give the 'drive' to procreate, plus the will-power and instinct for survival.

THE BLADDER

The Bladder is intimately involved with the Kidneys in transforming fluids into urine. It then stores urine and in due course excretes it from the body. The Oriental view of Bladder function is therefore similar to that of Western medicine.

The Bladder Channel runs parallel to the vertebral column, in very close proximity to the roots of both the peripheral nerves and the autonomic nervous system, thereby having a strong influence upon them.

THE LUNGS

The Lungs extract *Ki* from air, which combines with *Ki* from food. They subsequently send this *Ki* through the Channels to energise all the physiological processes of the body. The Lungs also disperse Ki under the skin to provide the body's outer defensive layer, which protects from pathogenic organisms and extreme weather conditions such as cold.

Because the nose is the gateway of the breath, the nose, and therefore smell, is controlled by the Lungs.

Physiologically, the Lungs' energy helps to feel sensations and 'reality' by enabling people to experience 'now', in the way that a child is always much focused in the present.

THE LARGE INTESTINE

The function of the Large Intestine is to receive the residue of food and drink from the Small Intestine, re-absorb some of the fluids, and excrete the remains as stools (the same as in Western physiology).

THE SPLEEN

The Spleen refers to the entire digestive function and therefore the extraction of nutrients and the resultant production of blood. The spleen as an anatomical organ in the Western sense has relatively little to do with this function.

The Spleen ensures the strength and development of muscles by extracting nourishment from food and transporting it to the muscles and all other body parts, especially the limbs. It is because food passes the lips in the first stage of digestion that the lips are closely related to the Spleen, as is the mouth and therefore taste.

The Spleen is also responsible for preventing prolapses by 'holding up' organs and other body parts (expressed as 'rising *Ki*').

In the mental sphere, the Spleen influences thinking, analysing, concentrating and studying, thus ensuring strong powers of reasoning and memory.

THE STOMACH

It is the Ki of the Stomach which ensures that food is sent down to the Small Intestine, rather than 'rebelling' upwards to cause belching, hiccups and vomiting.

THE HEART

The Heart governs the blood by giving it impetus to circulate around the body. As part of this function it ensures the health and strength of the blood vessels.

The tongue, which commands a very rich supply of blood, is controlled mainly by the Heart. The Heart therefore controls the sense of taste and affects speech.

Finally, it is the Heart which has the most general influences on the Mind, governing mental activity, emotions, consciousness, thinking and sleep.

THE HEART PROTECTOR

The Heart Protector is closely related to the Heart. It relates to the pericardium, which is the outer covering of the heart organ. It acts like a bodyguard, protecting the Heart from invasion by pathogens, temperature changes and emotional trauma.

Psychologically, the Heart energy influences one's relationship with oneself, whereas the Heart Protector influences the way one relates to others, especially in close relationships.

THE SMALL INTESTINE

The Small Intestine receives food and drink from the Stomach and separates the nutritious part from the waste component. This process of selection or discrimination is mirrored on the mental level in so far as the Small Intestine gives the clarity of mind to make decisions. These functions are often expressed as 'separating the pure from the impure'.

THE TRIPLE HEATER

The Triple Heater is the only 'Organ' which does not equate with a physical organ. Its function is that of a catalyst, regulating the functions or Organs in three distinct areas of the body. The thorax is known as the Upper Heater, which gives impetus to the Lungs' function of distributing body fluids. The Middle Heater is between the diaphragm and the navel, facilitating digestion and the transportation of nutrients. The Lower Heater is the area below the navel, assisting the separation and excretion of fluids. The Triple Heater is therefore concerned with regulating the free passage of body fluids between these three regions.

The Triple Heater also distributes the strength or *Ki* generated in the belly to the Organs, and the periphery of the body, thereby helping to protect the body. It also helps to warm and protect the physical organs.

THE LIVER

The Liver ensures that *Ki* flows smoothly through the body. In addition, it stores much of the blood during rest, and releases it during physical activity, ensuring the nourishment of the body, especially the joints, sinews, eyes and nails.

On the mental sphere, the Liver gives the capacity for vision and planning. Unclear vision leads to bad planning and can result in anger, the emotion associated with the Liver.

THE GALL BLADDER

The Gall Bladder is very closely related to the Liver in function, in that it helps the Liver to smooth the flow of *Ki*. As a physical structure, the Gall Bladder stores and excretes bile, just as we know from Western physiology.

Psychologically, the Gall Bladder complements the Liver's 'plans' by giving the courage and initiative to make decisions.

The Shiatsu therapist will understand the functions of the Organs from the Oriental point of view and from the Western point of view. He or she will also understand the pathology of Organ dysfunction from an Oriental medical viewpoint (to describe Oriental medical pathology is outside the scope of this chapter). Therefore, specific treatment strategies can be formulated based around which *Ki* Channels and *Tsubo* act to restore the *Yin–Yang* imbalance of any given pathology.

Another way in which the Shiatsu therapist can help alleviate illness and restore *Yin–Yang* balance is by infusing the Shiatsu treatment with the qualities that are lacking in the patient. For example, nurturing and support are qualities of the earth Element (Spleen and Stomach Channels and Organs). If a person has been denied physical and emotional nourishment, or has lacked support from family or peers, then the digestive functions will deteriorate. Shiatsu given with extra physical connection and support will, in itself, strengthen the digestive functions. Similar approaches apply to all problems that may arise.

Who
needs Shiatsu?

Everybody can benefit from Shiatsu by a strengthening and balancing of their vitality. Nobody is in perfect harmony. However, a person does not have to be ill to receive Shiatsu. Even the most elementary Shiatsu is able to calm a wound-up person, loosen up the tense muscles and stiff joints, and strengthen the general level of vitality. Below are some examples of circumstances when Shiatsu can be particularly beneficial.

Shiatsu helps to

- increase energy levels;
- increase body awareness;
- relieve stress-related anxiety and tension;
- induce very deep relaxation;
- ease aches and pains;
- boost the immune system;
- treat common ailments;
- increase flexibility;
- heal sports and dance injuries;
- stabilise emotional and psychological conditions;
- relieve backache;
- improve posture;
- improve stamina;
- improve digestion;
- improve libido;
- treat menstrual problems;
- benefit a healthy pregnancy;
- ease childbirth;
- relieve headaches and migraines;
- harmonise the body, mind and spirit.

There are certain circumstances where Shiatsu may be limited in its effectiveness, purely because touch is difficult and inappropriate. The following list highlights these situations:

- *Acute fevers*: most people prefer to be left alone when aching and sweating from a fever.
- *Contagious diseases*: it is not appropriate to touch someone with a disease that can be acquired through touch, for obvious reasons.
- *Internal bleeding or blood clots*: if there is any suspicion of internal bleeding, Shiatsu should be avoided, because it encourages an increase in blood flow.
- *Touch phobia*: if someone dislikes being touched, Shiatsu will be difficult to accept.

There are other situations where certain parts of the body must be avoided during a Shiatsu session. In these situations, another area should be worked on, which, by association, benefits the area that cannot be touched. These situations include:

- *Severe skin problems*: psoriasis or eczema may be so severe that physical touch is too painful, and possibly damaging to the affected area of skin (although there is usually some part of the body that can be reached).
- *Severe burns, bruises or swellings*: burns, bruises and swellings are painful when pressure is applied to them.
- *Fracture sites and areas of acute muscle or ligament injury*: broken bones and torn ligaments should not be touched directly.
- *Cuts, local inflammation and infections*: direct pressure would be painful.
- *Twisted intestines*: a twist in the intestines could easily become strangulated, thereby obstructing its own blood supply. It is conceivable that Shiatsu to the abdomen might strangulate an existing twist.
- *Varicose veins*: direct pressure upon varicose veins is very painful and likely to cause damage to them. However, Shiatsu elsewhere can, to some extent, be of benefit in relieving the problem.
- *During pregnancy*: Shiatsu can be both very relaxing and very invigorating during pregnancy. However, certain pressure points can have a deleterious effect by increasing the risk of miscarriage. The lower leg is particularly rich in these contra-indicated points. For this reason, giving Shiatsu to the lower leg should be avoided altogether, except perhaps, for some gentle work on the feet.

Shiatsu, by definition, requires actual physical contact. However, it is sometimes argued that techniques which use the heat radiating from the hands, but which do not make actual physical contact, can be considered supplementary Shiatsu techniques. These techniques are clearly not restricted in the contra-indicated circumstances listed above. Radiating heat from the palms is called *Hoshino* therapy. By rubbing the hands briskly together energy is created which can be transmitted at a distance.

Shiatsu is not a panacea, but giving and receiving human touch fulfils a deep need in most people. *Ki* is shared through touch. By keeping each other's *Ki* Channels open, much ill health can be reduced and prevented, and peace is spread around those who practise Shiatsu.

Reference

1. C. Jarmey and G. Mojay, **Shiatsu, the Complete Guide,** *London: Thorsons,* 1991.

Further Reading

C. Jarmey and J. Tindall, **Acupressure for Common Ailments,** *London: Gaia Books,* 1991.

C. Jarmey, Thorsons' **Introductory Guide to Shiatsu,** *London: Thorsons,* 1992.

S. Masunaga, **Zen Shiatsu,** *New York: Japan Publications,* 1971.

D.F. Rankin-Box (ed.), **Complementary Health Therapies: A Guide for Nurses,** *Beckenham: Croom Helm,* 1988.

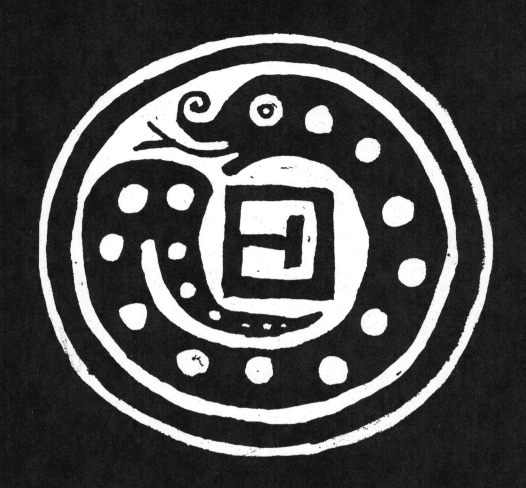

8

ACUPUNCTURE AND
TRADITIONAL CHINESE MEDICINE

Geoffrey Wadlow

Definition

Acupuncture is the insertion of fine needles into the skin and underlying tissues for therapeutic effect. Traditional Chinese Medicine (TCM) is the name given to the traditional medicine practised in China at the present day. It includes the following therapies: acupuncture, herbal medicine, massage, manipulation, dietary therapy and therapeutic exercise, all of which are practised according to the same basic underlying theoretical principles.

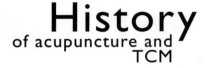

History
of acupuncture and
TCM

ACUPUNCTURE UP TO 1949

Chinese traditional medicine has always existed as a system of health care in its own right. One of its main strengths lies in its long history of development over the past 3,500 years.[1] The experience accumulated over this time has been recorded and refined, and provides a wealth of valuable theoretical and practical information about all levels of health care.

Chinese medicine has a developed and sophisticated intellectual tradition, supported by a large body of extant texts. Almost 3,000 medical titles are known to have been published in China between the Han dynasty (202 BC to AD 220) and the beginning of this century.[2] Other sources put the figure as high as 9,900.[3] The first Imperial medical college was probably established at the beginning of the Tang dynasty (AD 618–907),[4] as were medical colleges in provincial cities.[5]

Early origins

There are different theories concerning the origins of acupuncture. For instance, it is believed that the people of the Stone Age first used stone or bone needles to scrape the skin, lance abscesses and stimulate or massage painful points on the body, as well as for blood letting.[6] It was noticed that these points seemed to lie on definite pathways on the body surface, that the sensation of the needle was felt to pass along these pathways, and, that the above-mentioned points had distinct therapeutic effects on the body's physiology. Over time, this information was combined with basic internal anatomy and the theory of 'channels of energy' (*Jingluo*) was formed.[7]

Chapters 7 and 8 treat similar subjects. Readers may wish to compare the text and tables where appropriate.

The first written references to acupuncture occur in the second century BC in the classic known as the *Huang Di Nei Jing*.[8] This is the earliest extant textbook of medicine, and describes the basic principles of Chinese medicine, which have changed little to this day. There is every reason to believe that this work was the culmination of a long period of development, probably stretching back 5,000 years or more.

Commentaries and expositions of various branches and specialisations followed over the succeeding centuries, each adding further refinements and increasing the sum of practical knowledge available to later generations.[9] Paediatrics, gynaecology and obstetrics, orthopaedics, internal medicine, and the treatment of epidemic fevers, all have their place as separate disciplines within traditional medicine.

Decline

The process of development of acupuncture theory and practice continued unabated until the Qing dynasty (1644–1911), when it gradually fell into disfavour with the Imperial household. A general decline in standards of practice and scholarship culminated in the closing of the Imperial College of Medicine in Beijing. This, in turn, was exacerbated by the introduction of Western medicine, mainly through the activities of Christian missionaries.[10]

Traditional medicine generally, and acupuncture in particular, caught in a period of decline and low in confidence, were unable to withstand the onslaught of this intrusion. None the less, survival was ensured by the dependence of the rural population on its relative cheapness and easy availability. The missionaries were concentrated in the cities and did not penetrate deeply into the rural areas. Western medicine, when not provided by missionaries, was expensive and only readily available to the better-off. In addition, the fact that Chinese medicine was so rooted in Chinese culture meant that the depredations of the colonial period and the introduction of Western scientific thinking could not suppress it completely.

ACUPUNCTURE SINCE 1949

During the period of civil war and the Japanese invasion, traditional medicine continued to be extensively used in the countryside, in particular in those areas controlled by Communist Party forces, where Western medicines and medical skills were unavailable, or not affordable. While there were only 38,000 Western-trained doctors in

China in 1949, there were up to 276,000 traditional practitioners.[11]

Integration of TCM into the health-care system

It is therefore not surprising that on taking control of China in 1949, one of the first programmes initiated by the new government was the establishment of a health service in which traditional medicine was to be fully integrated, not as a branch of Western medicine, but as a medical system in its own right.[12] Western and traditional medicine were to exist as two parallel and integrated systems. Programmes were begun for the setting up of training colleges and hospitals solely devoted to the practice of traditional medicine. There are now twenty-four colleges of traditional medicine in China, with approximately 25,000 students on full-time, five-year courses. All cities and large towns have one or more hospitals of traditional medicine; most small towns have hospitals or clinics where both Western and traditional medicine are equally available.[13]

Thus, traditional medicine in China is not practised purely as an adjunct to 'modern' medicine, although each 'Western' hospital will have an acupuncture department. In hospitals where only traditional medicine is practised, in the form of acupuncture, herbal medicine and massage, Western diagnostic techniques are available and, if surgery or drug therapy is thought necessary, this will be used, sometimes in conjunction with traditional treatment.[14]

The potential of traditional medicine

The Chinese have built up a wide experience of the potential of their traditional medicine. The result is that the range of disorders treated by acupuncture and herbal medicine in China covers almost the whole spectrum of human disease. Broadly speaking, acupuncture is thought to be most effective in the treatment of functional disorders where serious organic change has not yet taken place.[15] Herbal medicine is used mainly in the treatment of disorders of the internal organs, including disorders involving organic change. Both are commonly used in the treatment of infectious diseases.[16]

The government continues to make significant funds available for research into acupuncture. The past thirty years have been marked by some major new advances in technique, in particular the development of acupuncture anaesthesia.[17] China has made much use of this in publicising acupuncture, along with new techniques for treating such disorders as deaf-mutism and paralysis resulting from stroke. In addition, much work has been done in researching theoretical and practical approaches mentioned in the classical texts of acupuncture. This has led to a refining of knowledge and an improvement in the effectiveness of treatment. Regular international symposia are held where the results of this extensive research are discussed.[18]

World Health Organisation and acupuncture

The Chinese Ministry of Health is also working closely with the World Health Organisation (WHO) in its programme 'Health for all by the year 2000', to promote the practice of acupuncture in the Third World, particularly in parts of Africa and South America, where it provides a cheap and viable alternative to expensive Western drugs or high-technology medicine. Based on the experience of the Chinese, in 1979 the WHO drew up a list of diseases considered to be amenable to acupuncture treatment.[19]

Table 8.1 WHO provisional list of diseases that lend themselves to acupuncture treatment

Upper respiratory tract
Acute sinusitis
Acute rhinitis
Common cold
Acute tonsillitis

Respiratory system
Acute bronchitis
Bronchial asthma

Disorders of the eye
Acute conjunctivitis
Central retinitis
Myopia (in children)
Cataract (without complications)

Disorders of the mouth
Toothache
Post-extraction pain
Gingivitis
Acute and chronic pharyngitis

Gastro-intestinal system
Spasms of oesophagus and cardia
Hiccough
Acute and chronic gastritis

Gastric hyperacidity
Chronic duodenal ulcer (pain relief)
Acute duodenal ulcer (without complications)
Acute bacillary dysentery
Constipation
Diarrhoea
Paralytic ileum

Neurological and musculo-skeletal disorders
Headache
Migraine
Trigeminal neuralgia
Facial palsy (early stage)
Pareses following stroke
Peripheral neuropathies
Sequelae of poliomyelitis (early stage)
Ménière's disease
Neurogenic bladder dysfunction
Nocturnal enuresis
Intercostal neuralgia
Cervicobrachial syndrome
'Frozen shoulder'
'Tennis elbow'
Sciatica
Low back pain
Osteoarthritis

ACUPUNCTURE OUTSIDE CHINA

Outside China, acupuncture has been traditionally practised in several East Asian countries. Japan, Korea and Vietnam have particular strong and developed traditions, originally transmitted from China at various periods during the first millennium AD. In addition, overseas Chinese communities, around the Pacific basin and elsewhere, took their traditional medicine with them during their migrations. As a result, acupuncture is practised widely throughout the whole of South-east Asia.

Acupuncture in the West

The 'opening up' of China in the nineteenth and first half of the twentieth century is not only brought Western medicine to China, but also allowed the spread of Chinese medicine to the West. A strong tradition developed in France in the early part of this century, particularly promoted by George Soulie de Mourant, whose writing, along with that of Chamfrault,[20] became the foundation for acupuncture teaching in the West.[21] Further development took place in the 1950s and 1960s, when acupuncture began to be established in other parts of Europe by doctors, physiotherapists and osteopaths who had gone to France to train. At the same time, Chinese practitioners who had settled in California began to train non-Chinese Americans and laid the foundation for rapid development in the whole of the United States during the 1970s and 1980s. Currently, acupuncture is practised in most of Europe, North America, Australia and New Zealand. Acupuncture was extensively used throughout the former USSR and in some parts of Eastern Europe, particularly in Hungary and Romania, having been introduced during the years of Sino-Soviet friendship in the 1950s. After the recent upheavals, the current situation in these countries is unknown.

International acupuncture training courses

As mentioned above, the Chinese themselves, during and since the Cultural Revolution, have, with the help of the WHO, encouraged the adoption of acupuncture and traditional medicine in Third World countries. This has been mainly achieved through WHO-sponsored short courses designed specifically for non-Chinese at the International Acupuncture Training Centres, set up in the late seventies in the Colleges of Traditional Chinese Medicine in Beijing, Nanjing and Shanghai.

However, the Chinese have also made these courses available to students and practitioners from Western countries, and this has greatly aided the development and spread of acupuncture in Europe, North and South America and Australasia. The Chinese have also begun to publish English translations of acupuncture and Traditional Chinese Medicine textbooks in order to facilitate this spread of knowledge.[22]

The current usage and status of acupuncture in the West

Acupuncture has become very popular as an 'alternative' form of treatment in the West. In his study of the views of young doctors about alternative medicine, Reilly found that acupuncture commanded the most interest.[23] The widespread research into, and publicity of, its analgesic properties means that acupuncture is often sought by those suffering from intractable, painful syndromes.[24] Thus it is frequently used, for example, in the treatment of arthritis. There has also been publicity about its role in combating addictions, such as heroin,[25] Valium and cigarette smoking. However, these uses do not represent the full potential of Traditional Chinese Medicine as it is used in China, as evidenced above.

Acupuncture
in the United Kingdom

Acupuncture has only been practised in the United Kingdom on a significant scale during the last twenty-five years. Prior to this it had been practised by a few isolated individuals, and by members of the Chinese community, although the first record of its use in Britain occurs in the eighteenth century. Dr Felix Mann can probably be credited with laying the foundations of acupuncture practice in the United Kingdom with the publication of the first modern expositions of acupuncture to be published in English.[26]

There are two main groups of practitioners in the United Kingdom at present: on the one hand, 'traditional' acupuncturists and, on the other hand, doctors, dentists, physiotherapists and midwives, who mainly utilise acupuncture for pain relief.

'TRADITIONAL' ACUPUNCTURE

'Traditional' acupuncturists, who practise according to differing interpretations of traditional Chinese medical theory, all use acupuncture as a complete therapeutic modality to treat a wide range of disorders. Their training generally extends for three years. The majority are not medically qualified, although their training includes Western anatomy, physiology, pathology and medicine.

The term 'traditional acupuncture' covers a range of meanings in the acupuncture profession. However, the underlying theoretical systems by which practitioners diagnose and the principles on which they base their treatment, are common to all (see 'Mode of Action' below).

Scope of treatment

Traditional acupuncturists treat mainly chronic illnesses. This is because, for many patients, acupuncture is a treatment of last resort, orthodox treatment having been unable to help them. Some seek acupuncture treatment as an alternative to drug therapy, particularly where long-term prescription is the only orthodox treatment on offer. In most cases patients have already consulted their orthodox practitioner. According to Thomas *et al.* 'Non-orthodox treatment . . . [is] used most frequently as a supplement to orthodox medicine'.[27] A small minority of patients will use traditional Chinese medicine as their first choice in treatment – for instance, consulting a practitioner for acute minor ailments. However, this is usually after having experienced the beneficial effects of treatment for a previous chronic disorder.

Probably the most commonly treated disorders are those where the origin is related to physical or emotional stress. Dysfunctions of the major bodily systems, digestive, respiratory, circulatory, reproductive, urinary, endocrine and musculo-skeletal, are all commonly treated as they are in China.[28] This particularly applies to conditions where an orthodox diagnosis is unable to identify any pathological or organic changes, although even disorders where there are pathological or organic changes may be amenable to treatment.

NHS versus private practice

The difference in approach to acupuncture between 'traditional' and non-traditional practitioners is mirrored in the way treatment is offered. 'Traditional' acupuncture is almost exclusively practised in the private sector because 'traditional' acupuncturists generally are not members of a state registered profession and thus are not qualified to work within the NHS. As most of those who offer acupuncture for pain relief do work within the NHS, they are able to offer this treatment free of charge.

ACUPUNCTURE FOR PAIN RELIEF

The use of acupuncture for pain relief by the orthodox professions has grown dramatically in the last ten years. This has mainly involved doctors (specifically, anaesthetists and GPs), dentists, physiotherapists and midwives. Many hospitals have established pain clinics and have experimented with the use of acupuncture analgesia. In addition, following recent research,[29,30] increasing numbers of GPs have begun to use acupuncture in their surgeries for the treatment of common chronic ailments such as asthma.

Those who use acupuncture primarily for the relief of pain do not normally subscribe to its traditional theoretical principles. Training reflects this, and is usually much shorter than for 'traditional' acupuncturists, ranging in length from two weekends to six to eight weekends over six months. Most of the 'traditional' approach is omitted from these courses, which concentrate on the use of acupuncture as an additional technique in the treatment of pain.

The value
of acupuncture

The Chinese see the value of acupuncture as threefold. Firstly, it treats disorders for which other forms of treatment are not as effective; for example, acute back sprain. Secondly, it does not produce the side effects often associated with orthodox treatment regimes. Thirdly, it has a low cost.[31]

In the West there is still scepticism about acupuncture's mode of action. The scientific and medical community find it difficult to come to terms with traditional Chinese medical theory, while at least acupuncture's analgesic effects can partially be explained scientifically within the Western orthodox medical model. Thus, within the medical mainstream, acupuncture's role in treating pain is seen as its most valuable and usable contribution. This is reinforced by the almost complete absence of side effects from treatment.

As mentioned above, other aspects of acupuncture's therapeutic potential are beginning to be recognised. Amongst those, such as GPs, who accept that acupuncture, on a pragmatic level, does have something positive to offer their patients, there is an increasing willingness to consider providing treatment or to refer to a 'traditional' practitioner.

Training
of acupuncturists

Until recently, the education of 'traditional' acupuncturists in the United Kingdom had always been a part-time activity, reflecting the nature of the intake to the schools, which was mainly by mature people undertaking a career change, or existing health-care professionals, both orthodox and 'alternative' or complementary, undertaking additional training. A higher standard of training is now generally accepted as being necessary, and all the schools of acupuncture in the United Kingdom are in the process of expanding their courses, some to full-time status. Training lasts for three years and includes anatomy, physiology, pathology and diagnosis.

The Council for Acupuncture, in conjunction with the Council for Complementary and Alternative Medicine, has now established an independent body, the British Acupuncture Accreditation Board, to oversee training standards and accredit schools and colleges where acupuncture is taught.

A variety of courses exist for medical practitioners, nurses and physiotherapists wishing to study acupuncture, with courses ranging in length from two weekends to two years part-time.

Mode
of action TRADITIONAL AND MODERN THEORIES

There are broadly two explanations of how acupuncture works. On the one hand, there is the explanation based on traditional Chinese medical theory, which is in turn based on concepts of health and disease developed many centuries ago, though arguably still relevant today. On the other hand, there is the explanation based on modern scientific theories of the body's physiological functioning. Because the modern theories will be developed below (see 'Research'), the discussion here is confined to the traditional Chinese theories and explanations.

INTRODUCTION TO TRADITIONAL CHINESE MEDICAL THEORY

Traditional medical theory looks at the health of a person in the widest possible context. This includes lifestyle, environmental factors and emotional and spiritual factors. As will be further explained below, traditional medical theory does not make a distinction between the spiritual, mental, emotional and physical aspects of a person, which are expressed through the concept of *Qi* (pronounced 'chee') or 'vital force'.

Traditional Chinese medical theory postulates that good health is essentially a question of a healthy internal environment. The body's ability to resist disease is based on this. Chinese medical theory has developed theories of disease causation which go some way to explaining why it is that some people, in apparently similar circumstances, are for instance, affected by infectious diseases and some are not; why some people develop cancer and others do not.

Chinese medical theory provides a practitioner with the tools to make reasonably accurate predictions about the nature and course of a disease based on the clinical application of 'the Four Diagnostic methods' (*Sizhen*). In addition, it has a complex system of symptom differentiation and pattern identification (*Bagang* or Eight Principle Patterns, *Qixuejinye*, *Jingluo*, *Zangfu*, as well as systems for differentiating acute fevers – *Liujing*, *Weiqiyingxue* and *Sanjiao*), making the process of diagnosis a skilled intellectual exercise.

The planning and execution of a treatment, once a diagnosis has been made and the aetiology and pathology determined, involves the formulation of a treatment principle and the translation of this into a prescription of acupuncture points. These points are chosen for their energetic effect on the channel and organ system and, therefore, on the *Qi* of the body. Additional points may be added to deal with specific symptoms or conditions. Treatment will vary according to the nature of the illness (for example, acute or chronic), as will frequency of application.

YIN–YANG AND THE FIVE PHASES (*WU XING*)

Yin–Yang and *Wu xing* are systems within traditional Chinese thought for categorising natural phenomena and understanding their relationship to one another. Both are founded on observation of the natural world and were the basis for two of the most important philosophical 'schools' in pre-twentieth-century China.[32] Both systems place the human being very much in the context of the natural world.

Chinese medicine views the relationship between the human being and nature as an integrated one. The human being and nature represent opposing parts of a unified integrity. At the same time, the human body is a miniature version of this enormous system – a miniature universe. Each person represents a unity of opposing parts.[33]

YIN–YANG

This is probably the most important concept in Chinese medicine. It informs most of medical theory in relation to physiology, pathology and differentiation of disease, as well as the determination of treatment principle.[34]

The Chinese character for *Yin* literally means 'the shady side of a hill', while *Yang* literally means 'the bright side of a hill'.[35] *Yin* and *Yang* are not opposites, as in 'black' and 'white'. Rather, they are the two complementary ends of a moving spectrum and, as such, are in constant flux. The classic example of this is 'day' and 'night', which exemplifies several aspects of *Yin–Yang* theory: thus the idea of 'day' is meaningless without the existence of 'night', while at the same time 'day' and 'night' transform one into the other in a continual process of change. In fact, 'day' and 'night' are relative to each other. So, in *Yin–Yang* theory, phenomena are categorised as being more *Yin* or more *Yang* in quality in relation to other phenomena. '*Yin* and *Yang* are relative terms. All phenomena have a *Yin* and a *Yang* aspect. There is no *Yin* without *Yang*, just as there is no (cold) without (heat).'[36] It is significant that in the terminology of medical Chinese the technical term used is *Yin–Yang* rather than '*Yin and Yang*', indicating that this is a single concept.

The *Yin–Yang* relationship in a healthy person could be said to be in a state of dynamic balance. For example, the activity of our waking hours is a more *Yang* state; sleep is a more *Yin* state. Both are needed for health. Within the day, however, there will be times of great activity (*Yang*) and other times of relative rest and quiet (*Yin*). To translate this into pathology, the person who never rests, in spite of a need to do so, would tend to exhaust their *Yang* energy. Disease in this case would be characterised by a relative excess of *Yin*, for example, feeling cold and tired, weak digestion, lethargy, a tendency to diarrhoea, a weak pulse and a pale and flabby tongue. The aim of treatment is to restore an harmonious balance by strengthening the *Yang*.

Table 8.2 *Yin–Yang*: basic correspondence of natural phenomena and the human body (see also Table 7.1 on page 133)

YIN	*YANG*
Natural phenomena	
softness	hardness
coldness	heat
wetness	dryness
darkness	lightness
paleness	redness
downward/inward movement	upward/outward movement
stasis	motility
Human body	
front	back
below waist	above waist
thorax/abdomen	limbs
interior	exterior/surface
Zangfu (organs)	*Jingluo* (channels)
Zang organs	*Fu* organs
Disease	
chronic illness	acute illness
mild symptoms	strong symptoms
`cold' symptoms	`hot' symptoms
`damp' symptoms	`dry' symptoms
under-activity	over-activity
weakness of *Qi* or *Yang*	weakness of *Blood* or *Yin*

Thus *Yin–Yang* theory is used to define the relationship between health and disease; it is used in differentiation of symptom and disease patterns and in diagnosis;[37] it is used to help categorise the site of disease, to identify the stage of development of a disease and, by extension, the prognosis. It also has a role in health maintenance and disease prevention.[38]

WU XING

Wu xing literally means 'five phases' or 'elements'. The *Wu xing* system attempts to categorise all phenomena into one of five categories: 'wood', 'fire', 'earth', 'metal' and 'water'. The system is based on the observation of seasonal changes through the year and the changes in the natural environment that occur from season to season. Each 'phase' or 'element' in the system corresponds to a season and has qualities ascribed to it which are analogous to that season (see Table 8.3).

In the *Wu xing* system, natural external conditions are related to the condition of the internal environment of the human body and, as such,

Table 8.3 *Wu xing* correspondences

	Wood	**Fire**	**Earth**	**Metal**	**Water**
Season	Spring	Summer	Late summer	Autumn	Winter
Climate	Wind	Heat	Damp	Dryness	Cold
Development	birth	growth	maturity	withdrawal	dormancy
Direction	East	South	Centre	West	North
Colour	green	red	yellow	white	black
Taste	sour	bitter	sweet	pungent	salty
Zang	Liver	Heart	Spleen	Lung	Kidney
Fu	Gall Bladder	Small Intestine	Stomach	Large Intestine	Urinary Bladder
Disposition	anger	excitement	worry	sadness	fear
Tissue	sinews	Blood Vessels	flesh	skin/body hair	bones
Sense organ	eyes	tongue	mouth	nose	ears

establish a primary connection between the human being and the external environment (for example, the seasons or weather conditions).

Just as each season follows the next in the yearly cycle, so this succession determines the relationship of one phase to the next. If each season occurs on time, and the normal weather conditions prevail, this will provide the right conditions for the next season. Each of the organs in Chinese medical theory is ascribed to one of the phases (see Table 8.3). Thus the seasonal relationships determine the relationship of one organ to another. If one organ is working in a normal, healthy way, this will enable the next organ in the cycle to do likewise. The internal organs have specific functions within the theory and do not represent the exact anatomical organ (see below: 'The Internal Organs').

These relationships, between seasons and organs in the body, are expressed in the form of cycles of 'support' and 'restraint' (see Figure 8.1). These cycles determine normal physiological relationships. Aberrations, for example, either insufficient support or the reversal of the restraint cycle, produce pathology.

The *Wu xing* system of correspondences is used diagnostically. For example, problems affecting the eyes are often associated with the Liver, and Gall Bladder organs and treatment will involve using points on the channels associated with them.

QI

In Chinese medical theory the health of a person is determined by a sufficient, balanced and uninterrupted flow of vital energy, or *Qi*, in the body. *Qi* ensures proper bodily function by keeping Blood and fluids circulating, by warming the body and by fighting disease. If the circulation of *Qi* is disrupted, becoming blocked or excessive or deficient, illness may occur, and this is described in terms of the *Yin* or *Yang* nature of the illness. Obstruction of the flow of *Qi* leads to pain.

Chinese medicine identifies two main types of energy in the body; the pre-natal *Qi* and the post-natal *Qi*. The pre-natal *Qi*, akin to a person's underlying constitution, is said to be derived from the parents of a child, its quality being determined by the health of the parents at conception. The post-natal *Qi*, which, being derived from the air and food, becomes operative after birth, is said be the *Qi* that flows in the channels (*Jingluo*) and regulates the proper functioning of the internal organs. The quality of people's lives, the food they eat and the air they breathe, all contribute to the quality of a person's *Qi*, thus playing an essential part in determining health and well-being.

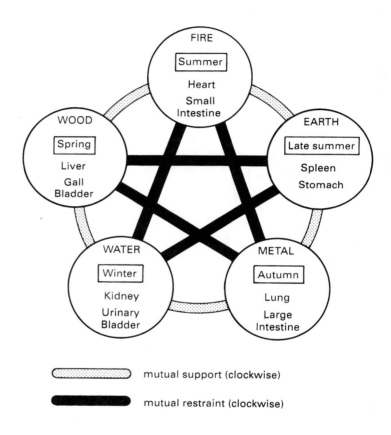

Figure 8.1   Wu xing: *relationship between the organs in Chinese medical theory*

THE CHANNEL SYSTEM, (*JINGLUO*) AND ACUPUNCTURE POINTS

The *Qi* of the body is said to flow along a network of clearly defined, though invisible, pathways, or Channels, on the body surface (*Jingluo*). These are the 'meridians' of acupuncture. These Channels connect the exterior of the body with the internal organs, the circulation of *Qi*

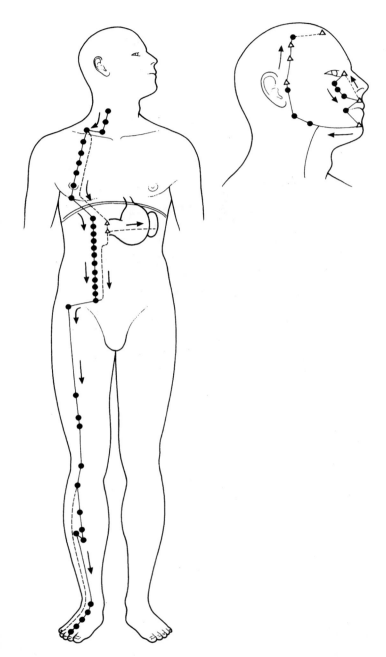

Figure 8.2   Stomach meridian of foot-yangming

through this interconnecting system being the means by which all the bodily functions are regulated. Thus the internal organs are said to be the means by which food and air are transformed into *Qi*, and by which the circulation of *Qi* is maintained and regulated. The Channel system is the means of distribution and circulation. Together, the Channels and organs form the 'anatomy' of Chinese medicine.

There are twelve main *Jingluo* which traverse the head, trunk, arms and legs at a superficial level on each side of the body. They are connected in a continuous circuit so that the *Qi* is said to flow through each channel in turn. Each has a deeper Channel connection to one of the internal organs (*Zangfu*) and is known by the name of that organ (see Figures 8.2–8.4). In addition, there are two channels following the anterior and posterior midlines. Secondary Channels interconnect the main channels, while others form a fine web over the most superficial layers of the flesh.

The acupuncture 'points' lie along the pathways of the main Channels. These points are categorised according to their effects in activating the *Qi* in the Channels and the internal organs. An intimate knowledge of the course of the Channels and the location of the points is essential for diagnosis and treatment. Needling these points activates the *Qi* to correct the pathology, either in the Channel itself, or possibly in another closely related Channel, or in the associated organs. Accurate diagnosis is essential for choosing the correct points if the best results from treatment are to be achieved. Points are used in 'prescriptions', on the basis that they will reinforce or mediate one another's actions and that this will be designed to enhance the overall therapeutic effect.

Traditionally, it has always been important for the success of treatment for a patient to feel sensation along the pathway of a channel when a point is needled. This sensation may be felt as numbness, distension, aching, soreness or heaviness.[39] Sharp pain is not considered of any beneficial therapeutic effect and usually means that the needle is in the wrong location, or that it has been inserted incorrectly. Much research has been carried out by the Chinese to investigate this phenomenon (see below). It is widely believed that the ancients discovered this and that by this means the pathways of the *Jingluo* were recognised.[40]

Disease will often manifest with symptoms along the course of the Channels, so they may be used as tools for diagnosis as well as treatment. The Channels are also the means by which disease may

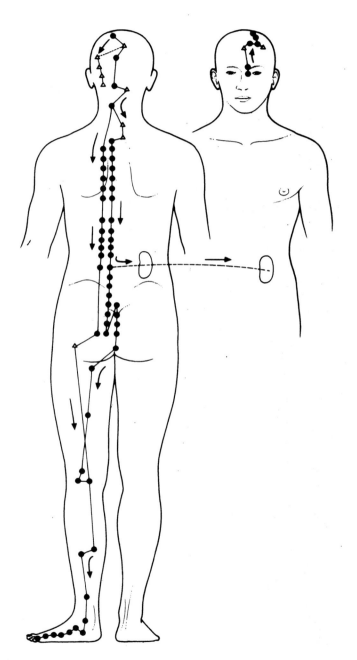

*Figure 8.3   Bladder meridian of foot-*taiyang

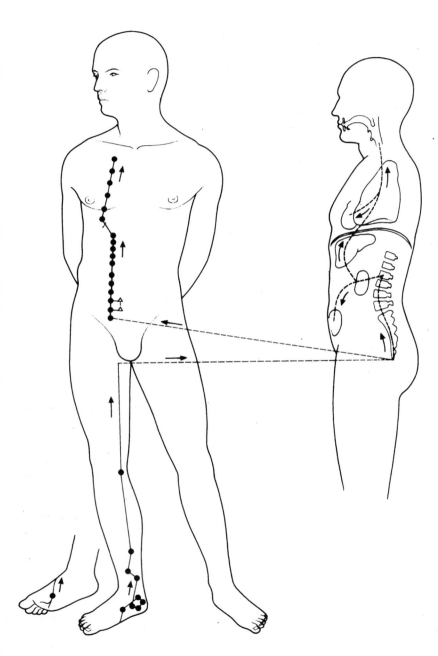

Figure 8.4   Kidney meridian of foot-shaoyin

be transmitted around the body. This transmission typically follows the relationships of the *Wu xing*, and it is possible for experienced practitioners with an understanding of this process to predict the course of a disease.

THE INTERNAL ORGANS (*ZANGFU*)

The internal organs described by Chinese medical theory have the same names as in orthodox medicine; namely, Heart, Lungs, Liver, Kidneys, Spleen and so on. However, rather than being strictly anatomical entities, the Chinese describe the organs in terms of their functions in relation to the production, regulation, circulation and storing of *Qi* (see Table 8.4).

The organs are divided into two groups: *Zang* and *Fu* which, joined together, make the collective noun, *Zangfu*, which means 'internal organs'. The *Zang* are the Liver, Heart, Spleen, Lung, Kidney and Pericardium; the *Fu* are the Gall Bladder, Small Intestine, *San Jiao* (organ peculiar to Chinese medicine which refers to specific energetic functions), Stomach, Large Intestine and Urinary Bladder. The *Zang* are said to 'store' *Qi*; they are known as 'solid' organs which, relative to the *Fu*, are considered to be more *Yin* in quality because of their functions. The *Fu* are known as the 'hollow' organs, and are responsible for 'transforming' food and fluids into the *Qi* which the *Zang* then store; because of their active function, the *Fu* are seen as more *Yang* in quality.[41] *Zang* and *Fu* are linked in pairs within the *Wu xing* system (see Figure 8.1) and also functionally.

Some of the functions of the organs described by Chinese medicine are similar to Western medicine, whereas some are radically different. An example is the Spleen, which in Chinese medicine is the organ which ensures that the whole of the digestive process operates effectively. The closest correlation in Western medicine is probably with the pancreas. In Chinese medicine, while the Stomach and Intestines transform food into *Qi*, it is the Spleen which regulates this transformation and ensures that the 'product' goes to the right places in the body. If the Spleen function is impaired, typical symptoms include abdominal pain, bloating, loss of appetite, loose stool or diarrhoea, cold extremities, tiredness, lethargy and, in extreme cases, weight loss and muscle wasting.[42]

In addition to specific functions, each organ is also closely associated with one of the sense organs and with particular areas of the body (see Table 8.4). These characteristics are used diagnostically, but are also important in treatment. For example, in eye problems, successful treatment will often depend on the acupuncturist including points on the Liver channel.

Table 8.4 Functions and characteristics of the main *Zang* in traditional Chinese medicine

	LIVER	HEART	SPLEEN	LUNG	KIDNEY
Wu xing	Wood	Fire	Earth	Metal	Water
Functions	Regulates volume of Blood in circulation; smoothes and regulates flow of *Qi* and Blood;	Controls blood circulation and blood vessels;	Responsible for the transformation of food into *Qi*; 'ascends' the *Qi*, i.e., holds the organs in place; maintains the integrity of the blood vessels;	Responsible for respiration and transformation of air into *Qi*; 'descends' the *Qi* (inspiration) and 'disperses' the *Qi* (circulation of protective *Qi* to body surface); role in water metabolism;	Stores 'constitutional' *Qi* (*Jing*) i.e. responsible for growth, reproduction and development; nourishes brain and spinal cord; role in maintaining bones, teeth, and blood; regulates water metabolism; aids lung in 'descending' *Qi*
Associations	Associated with the 'Soul' (*Hun*); energetic relationship with Urinary Bladder; physiological relationship with the nails, muscles and tendons, and eyes.	Associated with the functions of the mind, including the spirit' (*Shen*); energetic relationship with Small Intestine; physiological relationship with the complexion and the tongue	Energetic relationship with Stomach; physiological relationship with the flesh, the limbs, the mouth and the lips	Associated with 'animal spirit' (*Po*); energetic relationship with Large Intestine; physiological relationship with skin, body hair, voice, nose and throat	Energetic relationship with Urinary Bladder; physiological relationship with lumbar region, hair of head.

AETIOLOGICAL FACTORS

There are three main reasons why the circulation of *Qi* may become disrupted: internal, or emotional, disturbances; external, or climatic, factors; and imbalances in diet, lifestyle, or over-work or stress, and various miscellaneous factors detailed below.

Table 8.5 Aetiological factors and their effects[43]

	Aetiological factor	Effect
External (mainly affect *Jingluo*)	Wind	Symptoms arise suddenly and change rapidly:
	Summer-Heat, Fire	fever, thirst, sweating,
	Damp	turbid, sticky discharges,
	Dryness	dry mouth, dry skin,
	Cold	pain, watery discharges
Internal (mainly affect *Zangfu*)	Anger	Makes *Qi* rise; affects Liver
	Excitement	slows *Qi* down; affects Heart
	Worry	'knots' the *Qi*; affects Spleen
	Sadness	'dissolves' the *Qi*; affects Lung
	Fear	makes *Qi* descend; affects Kidney
	Fright	'scatters' the *Qi*; affects Heart and Kidney
General	Constitution: weak or compromised before, at or, since, birth.	Most likely to affect the Kidney, but can affect any organ.
	Diet: poor quality of food; irregular intake of food; excess of one particular type of food, e.g., fried, or sweet.	Mainly affects Spleen and Stomach; excess of particular taste affects relevant organ according to *Wu Xing* correspondences.
	Activity/exercise: mental or physical over-work; excessive amount of exercise.	mainly affects Stomach, Spleen and Kidney
	Sex: excess sexual activity (men) and childbirth (women), according to health and constitution.	mainly affects Kidney
	Trauma: accidents; physical injury of any kind.	affects circulation of *Qi* in *Jingluo*
	Addictions: food, alcohol, smoking, social drugs.	depends on addiction
	Poison/parasites	depends on agent
	Iatrogenesis: including wrong treatment with herbal medicines	depends on treatment or drug involved

In Chinese medicine the emotional and psychological balance of a person is an integral part of well-being. Emotional disturbance affects the *Qi* as much as physical trauma and forms part of the diagnostic picture, as well as being seen as a causative factor in the disease process.

The experience of intense emotions over a prolonged period, or repressed expression of feelings, are both said to injure the internal organs by disrupting their normal 'balanced' functioning.

Climatic factors – that is, excesses of Cold, Heat, Dampness, Dryness – are also seen as affecting the circulation and balance of Qi, predominantly in the Channels on the exterior of the body. Although in the West people are less exposed than they are in China to the vagaries of climate, such factors are still important in determining aetiology and, therefore, treatment. Diseases arising from climatic factors according to traditional diagnosis often correspond in Western medicine to diseases caused by viral or bacterial infection.

Consideration of a person's lifestyle and habits (such as eating patterns, work, smoking, alcohol, exercise and so on) plays a vital part in determining aetiology in disease and helping patients to understand their part in the healing process. It is also important to help patients to prevent further incidence of health problems.

Aetiology in Western medicine can be generalised into six areas: trauma, neoplastic, degenerative, auto-immune, genetics (constitution) and external pathogens. By contrast, Chinese medicine takes a more eclectic view of disease causation because it combines mental, emotional and physical functions in its view of physiology. Thus, an internal organ can be injured by emotional excesses, and mental disturbance can originate from organ dysfunction.

DIAGNOSIS AND DISEASE DIFFERENTIATION

During many centuries succeeding generations of Chinese doctors built up systems for differentiating diseases based on their observation of symptoms and signs. These systems group symptoms and signs into 'patterns of disharmony', and are the means by which practitioners make a diagnosis. A detailed knowledge and understanding of these patterns is necessary in order to make a diagnosis, especially as patients do not necessarily fit the patterns perfectly. In this respect, symptoms and signs are always read in context and may have different significance in different patients.

The first, most basic and most important, system for differentiation is called *Bagang* or Eight Principle Patterns. This underlies all other differentiations in Chinese medicine, as its categories determine the site and nature of the disease.

Table 8.6 Syndrome differentiation according to *Bagang*

Internal	External
Deficiency	Excess
Cold	Hot
Yin	Yang

These categories are further differentiated when applied to the bodily substances of *Qi*, Blood (*Xue*) and Body Fluids (*Jinye*).

Table 8.7 Syndrome differentiation according to *Qixuejinye*

Qi	deficiency of *Qi*
	stagnation of *Qi*
	collapse of *Qi*
	rebellious *Qi*
Xue (Blood)	deficiency of *Xue*
	stagnation of *Xue*
	heat in *Xue*
	haemorrhage
Jinye (Body Fluids)	deficiency of *Jinye*
	oedema
	Phlegm

If the disease is categorised as 'internal', then the differentiation according to the *Zangfu* is used; if 'external', then the differentiation according to the *Jingluo* is used. A simplified example of *Zangfu* differentiation is shown below.

Table 8.8 Differentiation of syndromes of the Heart[44]

Heart syndromes	Heart *Qi* deficiency
	Heart *Yang* deficiency
	Heart *Yang* collapse
	Heart *Xue* deficiency
	Heart *Yin* deficiency
	Heart Fire blazing
	Heart *Xue* stagnant
	Phlegm obstructing Heart
	Phlegm-Fire agitating Heart

In addition to the above, a differentiation may be made according to the *Wu xing*. There are also systems for differentiating acute fevers: *Liujing*, *Weiqiyingxue* and *Sanjiao*, although these latter systems are mainly used in conjunction with Chinese herbal medicine.

Specifically named diseases are also differentiated according to traditional pathological categories. Some examples are given in the table below.

Table 8.9 Differentiation of disease in Chinese medicine

Asthma[45]	Lung & Kidney deficiency
	Lung deficiency
	Phlegm-damp retention in Lung
	Liver *Qi* stagnation
Gastric/duodenal ulcer [46]	Liver & Stomach *Qi* stagnation
	Blood stasis
	Spleen & Stomach Cold & deficient
	Stomach Fire
	Stomach *Yin* deficiency
	Phlegm-Damp retention in Stomach
Dysmenorrhoea [47]	*Qi* & Blood stagnation
	Cold-Damp retention in Uterus
	Damp-Heat in Liver Channel
	Qi & Blood deficiency
	Liver & Kidney deficiency

These systems of differentiation give the practitioner a wide scope in the treatment of a variety of diseases. Modern Chinese practitioners tend to use a combination of all these or use the system most appropriate to the patient and the disease in question. Practitioners of traditional Chinese medicine in the United Kingdom who have trained in China or trained at schools following the Chinese approach, also do this. Other traditional practitioners tend to concentrate on one or other system exclusively; for example, the *Wu xing* system of differentiation.

DIAGNOSTIC METHODS

There are four diagnostic methods in Chinese medicine, known as *Sizhen*: 'asking', 'looking', 'palpating' and 'listening/smelling'. Each has an important place in the process of reaching a diagnosis, 'asking' or questioning the patient having a primary place, as the information gleaned from this method allows the appropriate use and interpretation of the other three diagnostic methods.

Examination of the patient's tongue and pulse are key elements in the diagnostic process. They give the practitioner information about the condition of the person's *Qi* and of the internal organs. In particular, palpation of the radial pulse at the wrist has been developed into a complex and skilled method of diagnosis. As such, interpretations of pulse quality are made in the context of the other findings obtained by the other diagnostic methods.

There are twenty-eight pulse qualities described in the classical texts; the radial pulse is divided into three positions and each position has three depths. The different positions are related to specific organs (*Zangfu*), or to parts of the body, according to context. The different depths relate to the energetic level to which a disease has penetrated, or from which it originates.[48]

The tongue also has an important place in traditional diagnosis. The body of the tongue and the coating are said to indicate the condition of the Heart and the Stomach, respectively. However, both can be applied more generally to the overall condition of the person as well as the condition of specific organs (see Figure 8.6). Shape, size, colour and texture of the tongue body are all taken into account, as is the colour, thickness and texture of the tongue coating.[49]

The diagnostic methods of Chinese medicine enable the practitioner to make a diagnosis based on the 'patterns of disharmony' described earlier. It is not possible to make a diagnosis based purely on Western diagnostic methods as these could not assess the disease process at the energetic level of *Qi*, *Jingluo* (Channels) or *Zangfu* (internal organs).

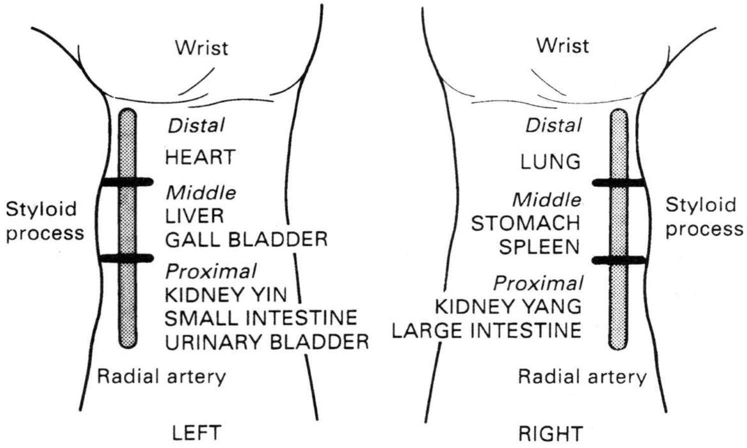

LEFT

Wrist
Distal — HEART
Styloid process
Middle — LIVER / GALL BLADDER
Proximal — KIDNEY YIN / SMALL INTESTINE / URINARY BLADDER
Radial artery

RIGHT

Wrist
Distal — LUNG
Styloid process
Middle — STOMACH / SPLEEN
Proximal — KIDNEY YANG / LARGE INTESTINE
Radial artery

Figure 8.5   Pulse positions at radial artery in relation to Zangfu

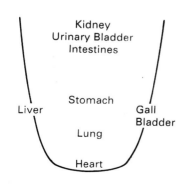

Kidney
Urinary Bladder
Intestines

Liver   Stomach   Gall Bladder

Lung

Heart

Figure 8.6   Areas of tongue in relation to Zangfu

Traditional
acupuncture treatment: techniques, usage, practical methods

FIRST CONSULTATION

At the first consultation, practitioners may spend anything from 15 minutes to 1½ hours talking and listening to the patient in order to reach a diagnosis. The length of time this interview takes is to some extent determined by the type of problem the patient presents. The interview focuses not just on the patients' physical symptoms and the history of the presenting problem, but also on their general physical and emotional condition, including aspects which they may not have thought immediately relevant. Their medical history is taken into account, as well as details of diet, work, lifestyle and social environment. Some practitioners pay more attention to physical symptoms, while others are more interested in the other aspects described above.

The tongue is examined, and the pulse is felt at both wrists. If the presenting problem is an 'external' musculo-skeletal disorder, for example, due to trauma, this aspect of diagnosis may not be used. Where relevant, a physical examination takes place, often concentrating on parts of the body which are tender on palpation, their location being of diagnostic value in determining the Channel or organ affected.

From all this information a diagnosis is made, and the practitioner explains this to the patient. Advice is given about diet, exercise and lifestyle, and herbs may be prescribed. If the practitioner is primarily an acupuncturist, the frequency and number of treatments needed is discussed.

TREATMENT PROCEDURE

The practitioner then asks the patient to lie on a couch, having exposed the parts of the body where acupuncture needles are to be inserted. The needles, which vary in length from 1.7 cm to 10 cm, are extremely fine (0.22 mm to 0.38 mm) and are solid (that is, not hollow). They are most commonly inserted in the forearms, hands, lower leg and feet, although there are frequently used acupuncture points on all parts of the body. The location of insertion usually depends on a combination of the site of the disorder and the way in which the practitioner wishes to influence the *Qi*. The depth of insertion varies from 1.7 cm to 7.5 cm, depending on the part of the body to be needled. Duration of insertion may be from a few seconds up to an hour, depending on the style of acupuncture being practised and the nature of the problem being treated.

The average time for retention of needles is 20 minutes, after which the needles are withdrawn. In some cases, the patient is then asked to lie in the prone position and further needles are inserted into the back. Care is always taken to avoid blood vessels and major organs, the anatomy of the points being an integral part of the training of traditional acupuncturists. Blood is rarely drawn and, if so, usually consists of a small drop. The need to eliminate the risk of cross-infection is taken very seriously by all practitioners, who are required by law to ensure that proper sterilisation of needles is carried out, or that pre-sterilised disposable needles are used.

The site of needling does not necessarily bear much relation to the disorder presented by the patient. This is exemplified by the use of points on the feet to treat conditions affecting the head, or the use of points on the upper lateral aspect of the lower leg to treat disorders of the digestion. The use of these points is determined by their therapeutic properties and the course of the Channel on which they lie.

The insertion of the needle should be painless, depending on the part of the body being needled, the degree to which the patient is relaxed and the skill of the practitioner. The latter generally reflects on the training of the practitioner; a well-trained acupuncturist will be able to insert a needle swiftly and painlessly. Generally, the patient experiences a mild pin-prick as the skin is pierced, followed by little or no sensation as the needle is inserted deeper. The practitioner may wish to obtain sensation around the needle or along the channel being needled. This may be a numb or distending sensation around the point, a tingling or electrical sensation, or possibly soreness.

OTHER METHODS OF TREATMENT

In certain conditions, the practitioner uses burning herbs to warm or stimulate certain points, which may or may not also be needled. This is called moxibustion, the herb used being the dried leaves of the common mugwort (*Artemisia vulgaris*), which are processed into a loose 'wool' or rolled into cigar-like sticks. Burning this herb has a particularly strong effect in warming and strengthening the body's *Qi* in conditions characterised by coldness and deficiency.

Other treatment techniques used by practitioners include cupping[50], massage (*Tuina*),[51] diet therapy,[52] exercise regimes and relaxation techniques[53]. All will be applied according to traditional diagnostic findings and can be useful and powerful additional tools in treatment.

TREATMENT PARAMETERS

Just as there are people who do not respond to drugs, so there are those who do not respond to acupuncture. Some diseases are very difficult to treat with acupuncture if they have progressed to the point where the body has become very weak. This is because acupuncture works by restoring energetic balance to the body and thus stimulates its healing powers. If the body is depleted, there are no reserves to call on and healing is very slow. Herbal medicine, diet therapy and *Qi gong* [53] are all used in this situation to rebuild strength and vitality.

There are no restrictions on who can receive treatment. Babies and children can be treated as successfully as adults, though the treatment of children is a specialised area in Chinese medicine and needs further training.[54] Women can be treated for complications of pregnancy without causing any harm to the mother or baby, though certain points have to be avoided if there is any likelihood of miscarriage.

Acupuncture can be combined with Western drug therapy, or can be used to eliminate dependence on drugs for some chronic conditions (in consultation with a prescribing physician). In this case the drugs will gradually be reduced as the effect of the acupuncture builds up. Treatment for chronic problems is usually once per week or fortnight. For acute problems it can be daily. The number of treatments depends entirely on the problem.

SIDE EFFECTS

Although most treatments will be completely free from side effects, some patients may experience pain due to poor needling technique. Others may experience symptoms due to inadvertent wrong diagnosis. This is particularly likely to happen where the practitioner has not been properly trained in traditional diagnosis and is therefore unable to make an informed and correct selection of point prescription.

Research,
including research in progress

A vast amount of research into acupuncture and traditional medicine is conducted in China.[55,56]. Much of this is criticised for poor research methodology and has largely been ignored or discounted in the West. However, many of the improvements in the technique and application of traditional medicine were based on this research, while many ancient techniques and prescriptions were clinically tested and verified as being beneficial or discarded.[57] This work needs to be duplicated in the West if traditional Chinese medicine is to advance.

Bensoussan gives a good overview of acupuncture research which falls into two very broad areas: research into the physiological effects of acupuncture, and research into the nature of the *Jingluo* (Channels).[58] These areas are subdivided as follows:

AREAS OF RESEARCH INTO THE PHYSIOLOGICAL EFFECTS OF ACUPUNCTURE

1 The analgesic effect of needling: in particular the use of acupuncture analgesia during surgery.
2 The regulatory effect of acupuncture: in particular, acupuncture's potential for effecting functional changes in the body's physiology – for instance, altering haemodynamics; also its potential for affecting the body's biochemistry, such as: the effects of varying the intensity and frequency of stimulation of needles during treatment; the effects of varying the number and frequency of treatments.

AREAS OF RESEARCH INTO NATURE OF THE *JINGLUO* (CHANNELS)

1 The anatomical relationships of the *Jingluo* and acupuncture points: the *Jingluo* and acupuncture points as a reflection of internal anatomy; the possible anatomical structure of *Jingluo*.
2 Propagated sensation along the *Jingluo*[59]: the therapeutic rationale behind propagated sensation; hormonal balance.
3 Acupuncture's potential for raising the immunity of the body, on the cellular level and on the humoral level; its effect on the reticulo-endothelial system; and, the anti-allergic effect of needling.
4 The sedative and psychological effect of needling; for instance, its use in the treatment of psychiatric disorders.
5 The relationship between electro-stimulation parameters and therapeutic results: this research has investigated the relative specificity of acupuncture points.
6 The electromagnetic properties of the *Jingluo* and acupuncture points.

HOW ACUPUNCTURE IS PERCEIVED BY SCIENCE AND MEDICINE

Basically, until the mode of action of acupuncture can be shown scientifically, large sections of the medical community will not accept its validity. However, as a practical therapeutic modality acupuncture is increasingly seen as valuable by the medical profession.[60]

There are differing views among scientists of the action of acupuncture in obtaining a therapeutic effect. These include theories about the nature of the Channels (*Jingluo*) and the acupuncture points in relation to the circulatory system, nerve pathways and dermatomes, their underlying anatomy, their bio-electric and electromagnetic properties.[61] Physiologically, acupuncture has been shown to have a regulatory effect, as well as an analgesic effect; to activate the body's immune system; and to have a sedative and psychologically calming effect.[62]

How acupuncture works is a continuing debate. There are three areas of investigation identified by Bensoussan:

1 Neural mediation, by which the effects of acupuncture are said to be transmitted via the nervous system.
2 Humoral mediation, by which acupuncture is said to affect the circulation within the blood and cerebrospinal fluid of neurotransmitters (for example, endorphins and enkephalins) and other hormones.
3 Bio-electric mediation, by which the channels are said to have electrical properties and that these properties can produce an effect on the neurological and humoral responses.[63]

In a concluding chapter to an exhaustive study of the research into acupuncture over recent years, Bensoussan advances the idea of a 'physiological learning process' as a possible mechanism. He writes:

> There is a need for more research, nevertheless the outcome of the thousands of clinical and experimental studies over the last three decades is that acupuncture stands firmly as a valid, viable and often preferable form of treatment, and certainly not just for pain relief.[64]

Summary

- Acupuncture, as part of traditional Chinese medicine, has a long and distinguished history as a therapeutic system for the treatment of human disease.
- A wide range of diseases are treated by acupuncture in China, where it exists as a system parallel and equal to modern 'Western' medicine.
- The practice of both 'traditional' acupuncture and acupuncture for pain relief has become widespread in the United Kingdom in the last twenty-five years.
- Acupuncture's strengths are: that it treats disorders for which other forms of treatment are not as effective; that it does not produce side effects; and that it has a low cost.
- Traditional medical theory looks at health in a wide context, including lifestyle, environmental factors and emotional and spiritual factors.
- The process of diagnosis and treatment formulation involved in traditional Chinese medicine is complex. It takes at least three years to train an acupuncturist properly.
- Research into acupuncture is extensive, but the physiological mechanism by which it works is unclear.

References

1   B. Hook (ed.) **The Cambridge Encyclopaedia of China**, *Cambridge: Cambridge University Press*, 1982; p. 139.

2   Ibid., p. 146.

3   Ki Sunu (trans.) **The Canon of Acupuncture – Huangti Nei Ching Ling Shu**, Vol 1 chaps 1–40, *Yuin University, Los Angeles, CA*, 1985; Foreword.

4   S. Palos, **The Chinese Art of Healing**, *New York: Bantam*, 1972; p. 8.

5   S.M. Hillier and J.A. Jewell, **Health Care and Traditional Medicine in China 1800–1982,** *London, Routledge & Kegan Paul*, 1983; p. 307

6   Hook, **The Cambridge Encyclopaedia of China**, p. 143.

7   Cheng Xinnong, **Chinese Acupuncture and Moxibustion,** *Beijing Foreign Languages Press*, 1987; p. 1.

8   The **Huang Di Nei Jing** or the 'Yellow Emperor's Canon of Internal Medicine' is divided into two books, the *Su Wen* and the *Ling shu*. Neither has been well translated in full. For a reasonable translation of part of this work see Ki Sunu (trans.) *The Canon of Acupuncture – Huangti Nei Ching Ling Shu*, Vol. 1 Chaps 1–40.

9   For an overview of the literature, see Appendix 1 in T.J. Kaptchuk, **Chinese Medicine – the Web that has no Weaver,** *London: Rider*, 1983.

10   This process is well documented in Hillier and Jewell, **Health Care and Traditional Medicine in China 1800–1982,** chap. 1.

11   N. Sivin (ed.), **Science, Medicine and Technology in East Asia**, Vol. 3, **Science and Medicine in 20th Century China: Research and Education,** Ann Arbor, MI: *Center for Chinese Studies, University of Michigan*, 1988; p. 246.

12   Hillier and Jewell, **Health Care and Traditional Medicine in China 1800–1982**, p. 314.

13   For an excellent account of the health care system in China, see Hillier and Jewell, **Health Care and Traditional Medicine in China 1800–1982.**

14   Based on personal experience during training in Jiangsu Provincial Hospital, Nanjing, in 1984–5 and 1986.

15   A. Bensoussan, **The Vital Meridian,** *Melbourne: Churchill Livingstone*, 1991; pp. 29–33.

16   Ibid., pp. 36–7.

17   For a comprehensive exposition of acupuncture anaesthesia, see S.T. Ho and L.K. Lu (trans.), **The Principles and Practical Use of Acupuncture Anaesthesia,** *Hong Kong: Medicine and Health Publishing Co.*, 1981.

18   For examples, see National Symposium of Acupuncture and Moxibustion and Acupuncture Anaesthesia, Beijing, 1979; also Second National Symposium on Acupuncture and Moxibustion and Acupuncture Anaesthesia, Beijing, 1984; All-China Society of Acupuncture and Moxibustion, Beijing.

19 R.H. Bannerman, Acupuncture: The WHO view, **World Health,** Dec. 1979, pp. 27–8.

20 A. Chamfrault, **Traité de Medicine Chinoise,** *Angoulême: Coquemard Press,* Vol. 1: 1954; Vol. II: 1957; Vol. III: 1959.

21 G. Soulie de Mourant, **L'Acuponcture Chinoise,** Paris: Jacques Lafitte, 1957.

22 Zhang Enqin (ed.), **A Practical English–Chinese Library of Traditional Chinese Medicine,** Vols 1–12, Shanghai: *Publishing House of Shanghai College of Traditional Chinese Medicine,* 1990.

23 D.T. Reilly, Young doctors' views on alternative medicine, **British Medical Journal,** 1983, 287: 337–9.

24 G. ter Riet, J. Kleijnen, and P. Knipschild, Acupuncture and chronic pain: a criteria-based meta-analysis, **Journal of Clinical Epidemiology,** 1990, 43, 11: 1191–9.

25 Bensoussan, **The Vital Meridian,** p. 34.

26 F. Mann, **Acupuncture: The Ancient Chinese Art of Healing,** *London: Heineman,* 1962; **The Meridians of Acupuncture,** *London: Heinemann,* 1964; **The Treatment of Disease by Acupuncture,** *London: Heinemann,* 1974.

27 K.J. Thomas, J. Carr, L. Westlake *et al.,* Use of non-orthodox and conventional health care in Great Britain, **British Medical Journal,** 1991, 302: 207–10.

28 For diseases commonly treated in China, see Xu Hengze, Ni Yitian, Liu Yaoquang, *et al.,* **Acupuncture Treatment of Common Diseases Based upon Differentiation of Syndromes,** *Beijing: The People's Medical Publishing House,* 1988.

29 K. Jobst, K. McPherson, V. Brown, *et al.,* Controlled trial of acupuncture for disabling breathlessness, **Lancet,** 1986, ii: 1416–19.

30 D. Aldridge and P. Pietroni, Clinical assessment of acupuncture in asthma therapy, **Journal of the Royal Society of Medicine,** 1987, 80: 222–4.

31 Hu Ximing, Vice-Minister of the Ministry of Public Health, People's Republic of China, in the Foreword to Cheng Xinnong, **Chinese Acupuncture and Moxibustion.**

32 Fung Yu Lan, **A Short History of Chinese Philosophy,** New York: The Free Press, 1966, pp. 30–1.

33 Liu Yanchi, **The Essential Book of Traditional Chinese Medicine,** New York: Columbia University Press, 1988; p. 9.

34 For a detailed discussion of this, see G. Maciocia, **The Foundations of Chinese Medicine,** *Edinburgh: Churchill Livingstone,* 1989; ch. 1.

35 Ibid., p. 2.

36 S. Mills (eds.) **Alternatives in Healing,** London: Macmillan, 1988; p. 8.

37 Ki Sunu (trans.), **The Canon of Acupuncture – Huangti Nei Ching Ling Shu,** Vol. 1, chaps 1–40, p. 11.

38 Ibid, p. 12.

39 Bensoussan, **The Vital Meridian**, p. 60.

40 Ibid., p. 60.

41 Maciocia, **The Foundations of Chinese Medicine**, p.68–9.

42 Ibid., pp. 89–93.

43 Ibid., pp. 127–41.

44 Ibid., pp. 201–13.

45 Xu Hengze, Ni Yitian, Liu Yaoquang, *et al.*, **Acupuncture Treatment of Common Diseases Based upon Differentiation of Syndromes**, p.23.

46 Kui Yang Bing, **The treatment of ulcer by acupuncture**, *Journal of Chinese Medicine,* 1987, 23: 17–19.

47 Xia Guicheng, Gou Huihong, Gu Yuehua *et al.*, **Concise Traditional Chinese Gynaecology**, *Nanjing: Jiangsu Science and Technology Publishing House*, 1987; pp. 104–11.

48 M. Porkert, **The Essentials of Chinese Diagnostics**, *Zurich: Chinese Medicine Publications Ltd*, 1983, pp. 129–54.

49 Ibid., pp. 193–253.

50 Cupping involves the use of small, usually glass, jars which are attached to the surface of the skin to cause local congestion. They are attached by heating the air in the glass to cause a vacuum which adheres the jar to the skin surface. See Cheng Xinnong (ed.), **Chinese Acupuncture and Moxibustion**, p. 346.

51 For an exposition of this subject, see Sun Chengnan (ed.), **Chinese Massage Therapy**, Jinan: Shandong Science and Technology Press, 1990.

52 See Zhang Enqin (ed.), **A Practical English–Chinese Library of Traditional Chinese Medicine, Vol.11, Chinese Medicated Diet.**

53 Exercise and relaxation therapies fall under the general category of **Qi gong** (literally, 'vital energy work'). They are used extensively for both rehabilitation, disease prevention, health maintenance, as well as for recreation: see Zhang Enqin (ed.), **A Practical English–Chinese Library of Traditional Chinese Medicine: Vol.1** *Qigong*.

54 For a detailed exposition of this subject, see J.P. Scott, **Acupuncture in the Treatment of Children**, Seattle: Eastland Press, 1991; see also Cao Jiming, Su Xinming, Cao Junqi, **Essentials of Traditional Chinese Paediatrics**, *Beijing: Foreign Languages Press*, 1990.

55 See Note 18.

56 For some examples of current research, see **Journal of Traditional Chinese Medicine**, Beijing, published quarterly in English.

57 Bensoussan, **The Vital Meridian** p. 6.

58 Ibid., chaps 2 and 3.

59 'Propagation of sensation along the channels' (PSC) is the phenomenon by which, when points are needled, it is possible to produce sensation along the length of the channel concerned. This has been shown to enhance the therapeutic effect of needling.

60 Reilly, **'Young doctors' views on alternative medicine.'**

61 Bensoussan, **The Vital Meridian**, chap. 3.

62 Ibid., chap. 2.

63 Ibid., p. 83.

64 Ibid., p. 132.

65 Available from the Council for Acupuncture, 179 Gloucester Place, London W1 6DX.

Regulatory Bodies

Most qualified practitioners of traditional Chinese medicine and acupuncture are members of one of the following professional bodies (the initials that practitioners use after their names are shown next to the name of the organisation):

British Acupuncture Association and Register – MBAcAR
Chung San Acupuncture Society – MCSAS
International Register of Oriental Medicine (UK) – MIROM
Register of Traditional Chinese Medicine – MRTCM
Traditional Acupuncture Society – MTAS

All these organisations are incorporated and have common Codes of Ethics and Practice, as well as the disciplinary procedures to enforce them. They are all members of the Council for Acupuncture, which publishes the 'Register of British Acupuncturists'.[65] Practitioners are allowed to advertise themselves and the clinics or surgeries where they practice in a limited way.

Registered medical practitioners using acupuncture may become members of the British Medical Acupuncture Society. For physiotherapists, there is a special interest group within the Chartered Society of Physiotherapists.

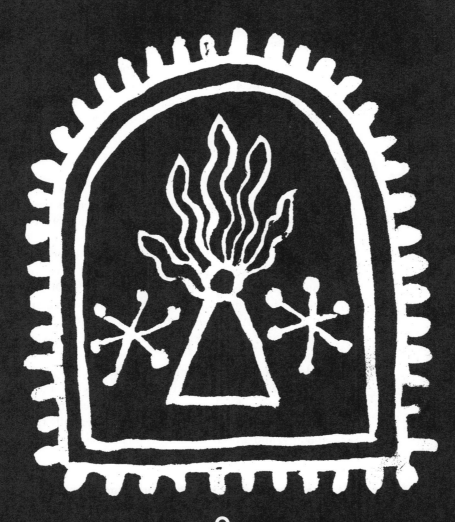

9

REFLEX ZONE THERAPY

Anne Lett

In reflex zone therapy the feet are palpated, and particular attention is given to those areas which are hypersensitive and to those which are insensitive to gentle probing, in order to alleviate pain and/or treat symptoms by stimulating the self-healing capacity of the body.

History

As far as is known, treatment of the feet has been used for thousands of years, mainly in Asian cultures, to promote well-being and to assist in healing. It was first described in the West as 'Zone Therapy' by Dr William Fitzgerald, an otolaryngologist, and Dr Edwin F. Bowers, in which they described how pressure applied to various parts of the body could be used as a means of relieving pain.[1] Dr Fitzgerald ascribed some of his findings to practices he had observed amongst several Indian tribes on the American continent, as well as to similar practices he had noticed on a visit to Central and Western Europe at the turn of the century.

In 1938 Mrs Eunice Ingham, an American masseuse, claimed that this method was equally effective when confined to the feet only. Since then, as the therapy has become more established and its practice more widespread, many people have been successfully treated with reflex zone therapy, and a body of knowledge has developed, enabling it to be used to greater effect.

Still widely practised in South and East Asian countries, the therapy has spread to the European world, and there are now few countries where it is not known. Many non-European countries do not have access to the drugs and machinery which are part of Western medicine, and rely on herbal and plant remedies as well as treatments that use local and available resources, which are usually built into the cultural pattern.

Benefits

With the increasing complexity of our highly technologically directed Western way of life, and the increasing potency and efficacy of drugs, some people have been found to benefit from simple forms of treatment as well as the more complicated ones. Reflex zone therapy may be practised as a complementary therapy on its own where this is appropriate, or in conjunction with modern allopathic medicine, although then the patient must remain under the care of the treating doctor.

As the therapy has become widely available, many people have found it to be an effective remedy for their complaints. As the only side effects so far observed (if the treatment is properly conducted) have been an increase in the excretory functions of the body, patients are prepared to tolerate the temporary inconvenience of such reactions if at the same time they begin to feel less sick.

Where it is possible to treat people with reflex zone therapy it has been noticed that drug dosages can be reduced or even sometimes eliminated. This would seem to be an advantage.

Current medical science does not accept, and there are as yet no tools for proving, the concept of energy fields in the body. Some doctors acknowledge the benefit of the therapy for their patients and are willing to prescribe it, or to monitor its use.

Practitioners and clients use reflex zone therapy because:

- it is not invasive as the client is not attached to any machine, and there is no perforation of the skin;
- it is inexpensive in equipment and resources, except that of the therapist's time;
- it may become an alternative to medication, which some people prefer;
- as drugs become increasingly expensive, cost may be reduced;
- the initial effect is of relaxation and 'winding down';
- the quality of sleep improves; consequently, people feel that they sleep more deeply, and are more alert when they are awake;
- pain and symptoms are relieved where the therapy is appropriately used;
- continuity of care between the client and a regular therapist is felt by both parties to be an advantage;
- many people, including the seriously ill, the terminally ill and the elderly, respond appreciatively to touch.

Code
of practice

Physiotherapy practice is governed by the Chartered Society of Physiotherapy. The Council of the Society has accepted the policy that the scope of practice should not be prescribed centrally by the Chartered Society of Physiotherapy. In future any practice which is recognised as appropriate to physiotherapy by a responsible body of opinion within the profession, should be regarded as within the scope of practice of a Chartered Physiotherapist, providing that she or he has undergone the training required by Rule 1 of the Rules of Professional Conduct.[2]

A special interest group for physiotherapists has been set up, and it is hoped that registered nurses and midwives will form their own special interest groups, which will allow the possibility of interdisciplinary co-operation under an umbrella group. The physiotherapists have taken the first step towards forming a regulatory body for themselves.

The National Consultative Council for Alternative and Complementary Therapies has set up a Council for Reflexology with the aim of drawing up standards and a Code of Conduct which will govern the practice of reflexology for those therapists whose practice is not governed by their professional training and bodies.

How
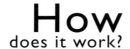
does it work?

No one has yet offered a satisfactory explanation of how the therapy works, although there are many theories. One frequently met is that the self-regenerating capacity of the body is stimulated by treatment. Another is that the many nerve endings in the feet, which may in the West be compressed as a result of unsuitable footwear, unused because of sedentary lifestyle and affected by poor nutrition, respond to the therapy as local blood supply is improved, and venous and lymphatic drainage is stimulated. In other countries where malnutrition and hard manual labour are the norm, these same nerve endings are affected differently. It must be remembered that small variations in balance because of the way we stand and move may also be responsible for changes in the tissue tonus and nerve endings in the feet.

It has also been postulated that endorphins are released with therapy, and that since they alleviate pain, that is why pain so often diminishes.

Yet peoples' feet do change with health and illness (bedsores are an example), in common with all other parts of the body. Swollen ankles may be the first sign of cardiovascular or renal disease of which people become aware. While it is not possible to make a diagnosis from observing or palpating the feet, they offer a surface for therapy in which the changes of improvement can be noted as well as those of deterioration.

A study 'The effect of reflex zone therapy compared with the effect of Flunarizin in patients with headache' was conducted by A. Lafuente, M. Noguera, C. Puy, A. Molins, F. Titus, and F. Sang in the neurological department of the Valle Hebron Hospital, Barcelona, Spain, in 1988, which concluded that reflex zone therapy and Flunarizin were equally effective in treating patients with headaches, reflex zone therapy having the advantage that there were fewer contra-indications and no side effects. A further study is currently under way in Barcelona.[3]

A normal healthy foot is warm, the tissue tonus is springy, leaving no colour change 30 seconds after light pressure has been applied, and the skin is elastic. On palpation of the foot, normal touch is experienced. If, on palpation, the patient feels pain, discomfort, or diminished or absent sensation, the reflex zone in that area is likely to be disordered, and needs to be treated for as long as these conditions persist.

If the practitioner experiences

- *fullness* of tissue tonus, so that it does not yield easily under the thumb;
- *weakness* of tissue tonus, so that the thumb falls too readily into the tissues;
- *crepitus*;
- *changes in skin colour* which persist for longer than 30 seconds after the thumb is withdrawn from the tissues, (although this may occur in some generalised diseases, and may be noticeable over the whole foot or body), then the reflex zone needs treatment.

When a reflex zone is found to be disordered – that is, if it is uncomfortable, painful, deficient in sensation or with abnormal tissue tonus – it usually indicates one of the following:

1 overtiredness, such as after night duty, or emotional strain;
2 the prodromal stage of an illness, such as discomfort in the zones of the nose and throat three or four days prior to a cold;
3 past illness, such as painful reflex zones to a tooth where there has been a past abscess, or in the reflex zone to the knee where there has been a previous injury;
4 a generalised illness involving the organ whose reflex zone is being palpated.

Very importantly, however, some patients presenting with symptoms also have local conditions of their feet, such as dropped metatarsal heads, fallen arches or calcaneal spurs, all of which may cause pain locally. Palpation of such areas is often uncomfortable, and while this may suggest that the reflex zone needs treatment, the discomfort may also be the result of the local injury.

It is, in general, worthwhile to treat the feet of people who have suffered a sprain or tendon injury in the past which has not healed normally. This delayed healing response may reflect a weakness in the underlying reflex zone and corresponding part of the body.

Individuals who have a longstanding generalised rheumatoid arthritis often have feet which are highly sensitive to touch over all areas of the feet, although this may not be the case if they have been on steroids for long periods. Seriously ill patients may also have hypersensitive feet in all areas, and this may also be less apparent when certain drugs are given in high doses or for long periods. In such instances palpating has to be done with great care until the feet become strong enough for normal touch, which may take weeks.

It is only the reflex zones to the nervous system which are found on the periosteum of the bones. For this reason palpation over bony surfaces should not be undertaken. Yet the bony structure of the foot provides a framework over which the reflex zones may be readily identified (see Plate 9.1, opposite page 47).

Assessment

A complete assessment of all the reflex zones of the feet is carried out at the first visit where this is possible. For details see Plate 9.1. Otherwise it may be spread over the first two or three sessions.

Any changes in the temperature of the feet, changes in skeletal structure, tissue tonus or skin, as well as reflex zones which are sensitive to touch are noted on the treatment card. The assessment consists of palpating the reflex zones of the feet in the following order:

1 *Head zones*, which are found on all four surfaces – dorsal, medial, plantar and lateral – of the ten toes. First the therapist will take the big toe at the interphalangeal joint between second and third fingers, holding with the other hand the head of the first metatarsal. Maintaining gentle traction, the big toe is gently rotated and counter-rotation is given with the other hand.

Beginning on the dorsum of the big toe, the reflex zones to the face are palpated, then on the lateral aspect of the big toe the reflex zones to the lateral musculature of the neck, the ear and mastoid are palpated. On the plantar aspect, first the tip of the big toe, representing the vault of the skull, the pad of the big toe representing the cerebrum, and then the cerebellum just above the joint space, as well as the pituitary gland, which is the highest point on the pad of the big toe, usually lying in the lateral half, are palpated. From the mid-line the therapist now tracks laterally across the base joint of the big toe to treat the musculature of the neck, which overlies the area of the proximal phalanx. The palpation of dorsal, medial, plantar and lateral aspects of all the remaining toes, first on one foot and then on the other, follows. Reflex zones to the teeth of the upper jaw are found on the medial and lateral aspects of the distal interphalangeal joint spaces, and those of the lower jaw on the medial and lateral aspects of the proximal interphalangeal joint spaces. Reflex zones to the eustachian tube lie at the base of the toes from the second to the fifth.

2 Musculo-skeletal system. After allowing the leg of the patient to fall into the outwardly rotated position, the reflex zones to the spine, which lie in the mid-line on the plantar aspect of the foot, are palpated, commencing at the interphalangeal joint space of the big toes. Tracking down the proximal phalanx of the big toe covers the area of the cervical spine. The dorsal spine lies alongside the first metatarsal bone, the lumbar spine along the cuneiform bone and the distal half of the navicular bone. The sacrum lies alongside the proximal half of the navicular bone and the distal half of the talus, and the coccyx has its reflex zones alongside the proximal half of the talus. Next, the reflex zone to the sternum, which lies over the first metatarsal bone on the dorsum of the foot, is palpated. The thoracic musculature lies in the spaces between all five metatarsal bones, and the shoulder joint has its reflex zones around the dorsal, lateral and plantar aspect of the head of the fifth metatarsal bone.

Reflex zones to the upper arm lie similarly on all three surfaces of the fifth metatarsal bone, and that of the elbow at the base of the fifth metatarsal. The musculature of the abdominal wall is palpated over the bridge formed by the tarsal bones. Those of the symphysis pubis lie in a crescent shape 180° underneath the internal malleolus, and those of the hip joint lie 180° underneath the external malleolus.

The reflex zones to the abductor muscles lie on the lateral aspect of the lower part of the fibula, and extend the length of the patient's hand's-breadth proximal to the highest point of the external malleolus. At this point is also to be found a reflex zone to the knee. The abductor muscles are palpated on the medial aspect of the lower part of the tibia.

3 *Heart*. Reflex zones to the heart are found over the distal half of metatarsal bones one and two on the left foot, and over the distal half of metatarsal bone one on the right, on both dorsal and plantar aspects.

4 *Lungs*. Reflex zones to the nose and mouth lie on the dorsum of the big toe, over the interphalangeal joint line. Those to the trachea lie in the space between metatarsal bone one and two on plantar and dorsal aspects, and the reflex zones to the lungs occupy the area over metatarsal bones two, three and four on the sole, and in the spaces between the second, third and fourth metatarsal bones on the dorsum. Tracing the arch where the texture of the foot changes from the sole to the ball of the foot follows the line of the diaphragm, and midway between metatarsals two and three, proximal to the heads of the metatarsals, lies the reflex zone to the solar plexus. A gentle sustained hold over this area has a calming effect on most people.

5 *Urinary system*. Reflex zones to the kidneys are found at the base of metatarsal bones two and three on the sole. Medial to this lies the reflex zone to the pelvi-ureteric junction, and those of the ureters lie medial to the tendon hallucis longus which is easily visible and palpable when the toe is dorsiflexed. The reflex zones to the bladder lie on the medial aspect of the heel, below the internal malleolus. Treating these areas will often obviate the need for catheterisation after surgery or delivery. It is helpful to treat the reflex zones to the solar plexus at the same time.

6 *Alimentary tract*. As already described, the reflex zones to the mouth are found on the dorsum of the big toe, below those of the nose, over the interphalangeal joint space. This area forms the naso-pharynx. Those to the oesophagus lie between metatarsal bones one and two on dorsum and sole, overlying those of the trachea. At the entrance to the stomach, the reflex zone to the cardia lies on the left foot, in the space between metatarsal bone one and two at the midpoint.

Reflex zones to the stomach are found on the proximal half of metatarsal bone one of left and right foot on the sole. On the right foot the reflex zone to the pylorus lies at the base of metatarsal bones one and two, where is also found the duodenal cap. The sphincter of Oddi and the duct of Wirschung lie on the sole just below the base of metatarsal two. The loops and coils of the small intestine lie beneath the tarsal bones in the arch of the foot. The ileo-caecal valve and the appendix are found on the sole of the right foot, where the calcaneum and cuboid bones meet, on the lateral half. The reflex zones of the large intestine lie beneath the cuboid and cuneiform bones on both feet, and those of the rectum and anus lie in the mid-line where the texture of the feet changes from the arch to the heel.

Reflex zones to the liver lie on the right foot, underneath the proximal third of metatarsal bones two, three, four and five, and that of the gall bladder lies towards the base of metatarsal bones three and four on the sole.

7 Lymphatic system. Lying in the webs between the toes are the reflex zones of the lymph nodes of the head and neck. Those of the tonsils lie on the dorsum of the big toe on the lateral border towards the base of the big toe. Reflex zones to the breasts extend across metatarsal bones two, three and four on the dorsum. (The tonus here is noticeably deficient within forty-eight hours of a mastectomy, and even though it may become puffy and fluid-filled thereafter, it will always feel less resistant to probing than normal tissue tonus).

The reflex zones to the axillary lymph nodes lie on the dorsal, lateral and plantar aspects of the feet below those of the shoulder joint, around the fifth metatarsal bone. That of the spleen lies on the plantar aspect of the left foot, beneath the base of metatarsal bones three, four and five. Those of the lymph nodes in the groin lie on the dorsum of the foot between the external and internal malleoli. The reflex zones of the lymphatic drainage of the pelvis lie on the medial and lateral aspects of the heels, and also on the plantar heel. Those of the lymphatic drainage of the thigh lie medially and laterally alongside the Achilles tendon, and extend about a hand's-breadth above the highest point of the malleolus. This area frequently becomes puffy when there are gynaecological disorders.

8 The endocrine system. The reflex zones to the pituitary gland lie on the plantar aspect of the big toe, at its highest point, and there is often a small protrusion here. The reflex zone to the thyroid gland lies at the base of the big toe on the dorsum, and extends over the whole of the head of metatarsal bone one and the proximal end of the proximal phalanx of the big toe on the plantar aspect. Those of the adrenal glands lie between metatarsal bones two and three, about one-third of the way distal to the bases.

Reflex zones to the head of the pancreas are found on the right foot, underneath the base of metatarsal bone one and its junction with the first cuneiform bone. Those of the body and tail of the pancreas lie on the left foot, underneath the bases of metatarsal bones one, two and three and the heads of the first, second and third cuneiform bones.

The reflex zones to the uterus and the prostate are found on the medial aspect of the heel, between the internal malleolus and the angle of the heel; and those of the ovaries and the lateral end of the inguinal canal lie on the lateral aspect of the heels, midway between the angle of the heel and the highest point of the internal malleolus. Further reflex zones to the pelvic organs lie on the plantar heel, beneath the calcaneum.

At the end of the assessment, the stroking movements are repeated, any changes in the temperature of the feet or the colour of the skin are noted, and the patient is left to rest quietly for twenty minutes, warmly covered.

Treatment

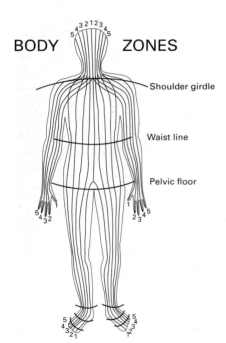

The ten longitudinal zones and three transverse zones

At the first assessment session and subsequent treatments it is assumed that there is an 'energy picture' of the head, neck and trunk on the feet. Every organ and structure is represented on the plantar and dorsal aspect, often lying over one another, as in the body.

The dorsum of the foot reflects the ventral surface of the body, the plantar surface of the foot reflects the dorsal or posterior surface of the body. By treating those organs which are not functioning as well as they might, an impulse is thought to be transmitted to the part of the body which is disordered, stimulating the healing process.

For the purposes of treatment, the body is divided into ten equal longitudinal zones, five on the left and five on the right. The right half of the body is reflected in the right foot and the left half of the body in the left foot. Body zones 1–5 lie on either side of the mid-line with body zone 5 being the most lateral.

Three transverse body zones correspond to the level of the shoulder girdle at the metatarso-phalangeal joint line; the level of the waist line where the metatarsal bones meet the cuneiform and cuboid bones; and the level of the pelvic floor, the hip joint and the symphysis pubis around the external and internal malleolus, respectively.

Technique

Lay your hand on any flat surface and notice how the thumb is rotated medially. This is the natural position of the hand for delivering therapy. The medial tip of the thumbs and the tips of the fingers are used to palpate the feet. It is easier to begin working with the thumbs before using all fingers, as the method when correctly learned by the thumb is then more easily transferred to the fingers.

The fingers of the hand are laid supportively on the dorsum of the

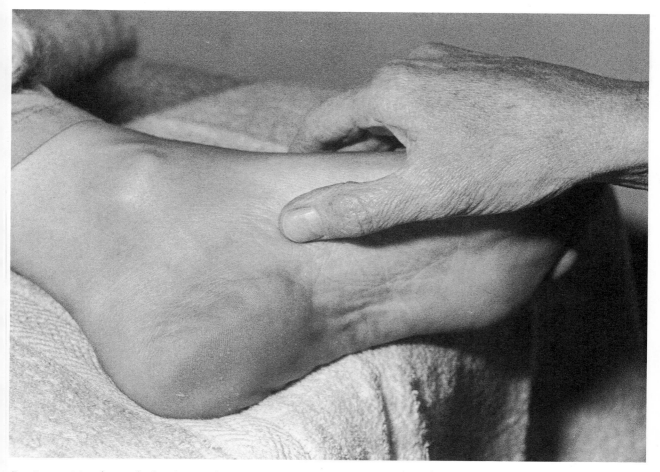

Resting position from which palpation begins

feet, without giving any counter-pressure, keeping the base joint of the thumb and that of the interphalangeal joint in a slightly flexed position. The thumb is allowed gently to probe the tissue tonus of the feet without permitting the flexion of the thumb to exceed 90 degrees, and only to deliver the probing pressure which the patient can comfortably bear. Now the muscle at the base joint of the thumb is allowed to relax. This allows the tip of the thumb to retract slowly from the tissues and come to rest on the surface of the skin. This movement is repeated, moving forwards or sideways in millimetre steps as the surface of the foot which it is wished to explore is palpated. The areas of your palpation where the patient feels changes in sensation or those where the tissue tonus is altered are noted.

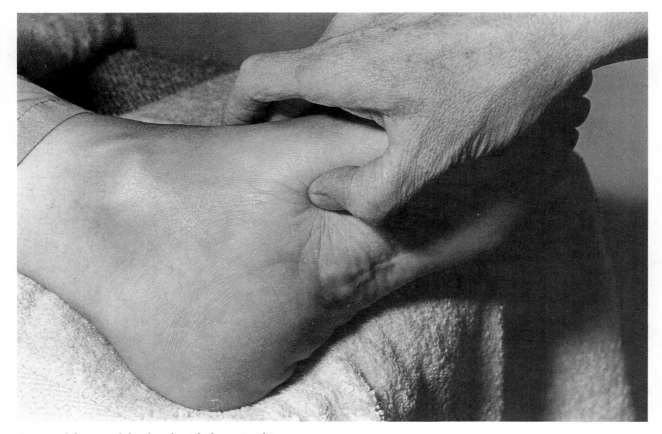

Increased flexion of the thumb with deeper probing

When working with the fingers, all the joints should be in slight flexion as probing takes place, the wrist held level and straight in order not to strain the joints. Work either with the thumb or the fingers so that pressure is not being applied to both surfaces of the feet.

The foot on which work is not being done should be covered at all times, otherwise it quickly feels cold, causing discomfort to the patient.

It is necessary that the practitioner allows the muscles at the base of the thumb to relax before withdrawing the tip of the thumb. If this is not done, the therapist's hands may become stiff and sore as undue strain is imposed on joints, and the therapy will be experienced as jabbing for the patient. For the same reason the joints should not be hyperextended for any length of time, and should not be kept in positions of pronation or supination whilst palpating.

This is the basic movement which the practitioner will use for the initial assessment and for all further treatment. As skill increases, variations will be introduced which are best learned in practical instruction. This basic movement may, however, be adapted to give first aid, when consistent, sustained pressure is applied to a reflex zone which is painful and corresponds to an area of the body where there is acute pain or limitation of movement.

For example, if someone is suffering acute lumbar pain, the reflex zones of the lumbar spine are probed to find the area which is most painful. The thumb then probes as deeply as the pain permits, and remains in position for 2 or 3 minutes until the pain in the area of the foot under the thumb lessens. This is often accompanied by relief of pain in the back. Similarly, the reflex zone to the solar plexus may be held firmly for someone who cannot sleep or has generalised pain. However, this is first aid and a temporary alleviation. The first aid hold should not be used to mask symptoms which should be investigated. In someone who is terminally ill, this sedation hold may be used as often as necessary for hiccups or nausea or pain.

POSITIONING OF THE PATIENT

Where possible the patient lies supine on a bed or couch of a comfortable height, with the feet about 1.3 cm from the end of the edge of the couch. The patient is supported with enough pillows to see the therapist's face. Thus the therapist is able to monitor the colour and expression of the patient's face and the rate and rhythm of the breathing. A small pillow or support under the knees of the patient will keep them flexed, and is advisable for the duration of the treatment and rest period only. A small towel under the feet is useful in case of sweating. Light and warm coverings, a warm room temperature and a restful atmosphere are also needed. The patient will be more comfortable if all constricting clothes are loosened.

POSITION OF THE THERAPIST

A chair, preferably without arms, or a stool of suitable height for the practitioner, is placed at the foot of the bed, so that the therapist can sit a forearm's length from the patient's feet. A relaxed shoulder girdle allows the arms to be held slightly away from the body, with the wrists held straight and slight flexion in all joints of fingers and thumbs. The back and neck will benefit from being held slightly erect. The therapist adopts a

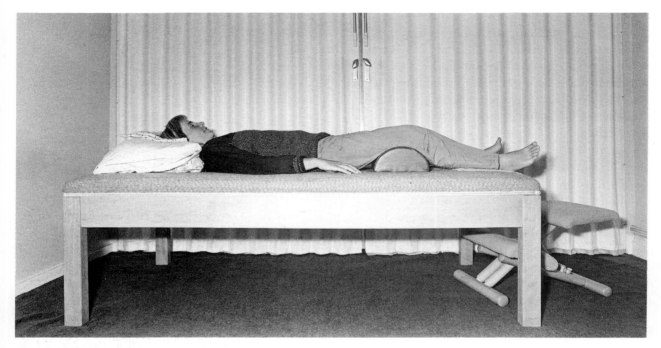

The position of the patient

comfortable sitting position with the knees in line with the hips and the feet firmly placed on the floor below the knees. This relaxed yet balanced posture allows the practitioner to observe the patient throughout, improves the respiratory capacity and gives no strain to the body.

Treatment

INSPECTION

The feet are carefully inspected before any palpation.

Temperature. The temperature of the feet, ankle and lower leg may be assessed by simultaneously passing the palms of the hand in one long downward stroke from knee to dorsal toes with one hand, and simultaneously from the ball of the foot towards midcalf with the other, keeping as close a contact with the skin as possible throughout the stroke. First one foot, then the other, are assessed for temperature, and the stroke may be repeated three or four times as it relaxes the patient.

Skeletal structure. The bony structures are observed, and any abnormalities such as hallux valgus, hammering of the toes or dropped arches are noted.

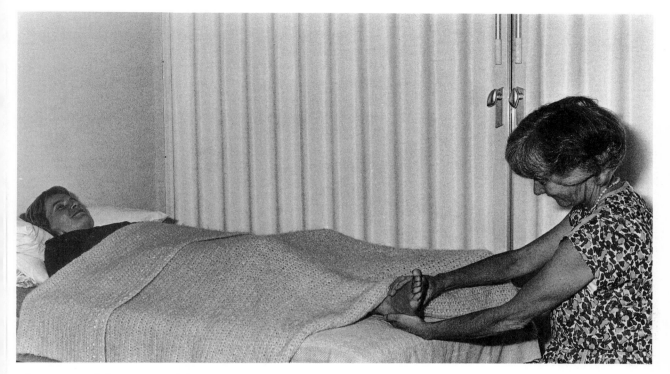

The position of the patient and therapist

Tissue tonus. The first look takes in the contour of the foot as a whole, noting any irregularities such as fullness or deficiency of tissue tonus in the ankles, lower calves, dorsum and sole.

The skin. Now the practitioner will look at the colour, transparency, elasticity and hydration of the skin, and at any areas of discoloration. Corns, calluses and fungal infections should also be noted, as well as the size and shape of each toenail. Persisting changes in colour and texture usually mean that the underlying reflex zone is not as healthy as it might be, and consequently also the organ to which it relates.

The practitioner will explain to the patient what is about to be done, and demonstrate how palpation is done on her or his own or the patient's hand. The practitioner will explain the probing of the surface of the foot, and ask the patient to report any discomfort or change in sensation as palpation is taking place. With more experience, the therapist is more able to rely on observation of changes in the tissue tonus. The patient, where able to do so, participates by saying what she or he is experiencing. Once the treatment has started, contact is maintained all the time with one foot or the other.

The feet are supported in a light hold, preferably with both hands, but not so tightly that the patient is unable to withdraw the foot if there is sudden discomfort. The feet are held in as natural a position as possible for the patient, and the weight of the hands should not rest on the feet.

No oils, talcum powder or implements are used as they mask the important reactions of cooling, sweating and changes in skin colour. If wished, or if the skin is dry, a little cream or oil may be applied at the end of the treatment with gentle, relaxing massage.

If the patient becomes restless, sweaty, cold or dry-mouthed, one or more of the harmonising measures may be used to restore him or her.

1 The palms of the hands are placed against the soles of the feet, reaching to the tips of the toes, and the feet are warmed by the close contact of the therapist's hands, without dorsiflexing the feet.

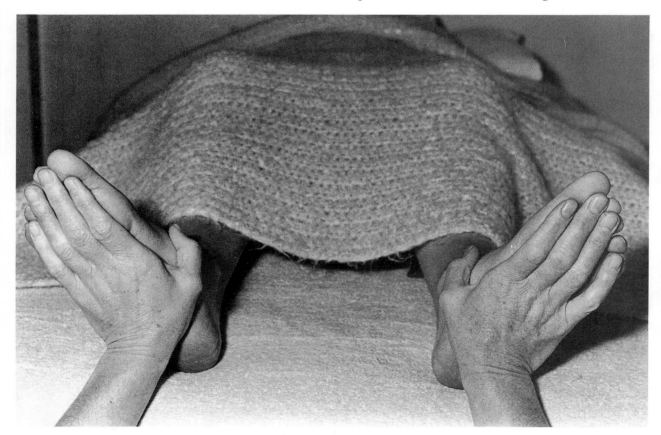

The palms of the hands support the soles of the feet

2 Both heels may be taken into the hands, keeping the fingers flat alongside the medial aspect of the heels. Gentle traction is applied to the heels as the patient breathes in, and released as the patient breathes out. On no account should the practitioner breathe in and out with the patient, but should maintain her or his own breathing rhythm.

3 Alternatively, the hands may be placed gently over the head of metatarsal bone one and the metatarso-phalangeal joint, and this area held for 20 to 30 seconds.

4 Another choice is for the therapist to place both thumbs in the reflex zone to the solar plexus and apply a little gentle pressure to these areas as the patient breathes in, which is released as the patient breathes out.

Any combination of these holds may be used until the feet are again warmed, the sweating has stopped or the restlessness has passed. The palpation may then be continued, but should the cooling, sweating, restlessness or dry mouth recur, the treatment is ended with effleurage strokes, which are long, even and gentle stroking movements in which one hand moves up the sole and inner aspect of the lower leg whilst the other hand moves simultaneously down the outer aspect of the leg towards the foot and over the dorsum. If the feet remain cold, give a warm footbath, and leave the patient warmly covered and resting under observation.

All the findings should be recorded accurately and in detail as soon as the treatment is finished.

If the feet remain cold, and signs of discomfort continue, the patient is given a warm footbath before being left to rest, and this is repeated four-hourly for as long as is necessary.

Since there are several possible causes for painful reflex zones, it is not possible at the first assessment to say why there are areas of discomfort. Remember that it is not possible to make a definitive diagnosis from your findings on the feet, as areas which were uncomfortable at one visit may not be so at the next.

Reactions

Before giving treatment, it is wise to inform the patient that there may be reactions, which usually take the form of change in bodily functions. When treating the very sick the therapist begins gently and lightly, the aim being to alleviate the most distressing symptoms – usually pain, breathlessness, nausea and restlessness – and not to provoke reactions which are too strong. If the patient or those in attendance on him or her are able to report any changes which take place, this is helpful to the therapist, and will help to decide the further pattern of treatment.

Reactions which may occur during a treatment session are:

- pallor;
- cooling of the feet;
- sweating, which usually appears first on the feet;
- dryness of the mouth;
- faster and shallower breathing.

At the first sign of any of these changes, the therapist will stop whatever she or he is doing, and, keeping contact with both feet, will use one or more of the harmonising measures already described. When the reactions cease, the treatment is restarted in another area of the feet. If they recur, the treatment is brought to an end with the effleurage strokes, a warm footbath is given if necessary, and the patient is left warmly covered and resting under observation.

Other reactions which may occur during treatment include change of expression, whether of tension or relaxation; general relaxation (usually visible in hand movements as the hands open and the arms fall to the side of the body); the breathing becomes deeper and more rhymthical; sighing or laughing. Some people and many children laugh nervously when they are anxious.

The therapist will watch the breathing of the patient at all times. As the patient becomes more relaxed, the breathing becomes deeper and slower. Faster, shallower respirations indicate that the patient is nervous or in pain, or that the treatment is causing discomfort.

Reactions which may follow treatment are:

A sense of relaxation.
Tiredness, usually after early sessions, and the patient will benefit from adequate rest in the early stages.
The urine may become more concentrated, with an acrid smell.
The bowels may become more active, with the stools being more bulky. These may also have a stronger smell than usual, and there may be more mucous and more flatulence.
The skin may perspire more freely, and occasionally there is a rash.
There may be increased catarrh, sputum or phlegm. This may change in colour, odour and consistency for a short time.
There may be an increase in vaginal and urethral discharges.
The patient may experience a headache during the early treatment

sessions. While this may at times be acute, it does not last longer than a few hours.

There may be an exacerbation of pain or of the original symptoms for which the patient is receiving treatment. (If the therapist is treating a seriously ill or dying patient only very gentle therapy, with frequent harmonising holds, will be given so as not to increase the distress of the patient.)

Menses may be heavier and earlier than usual.

There may be some change in appetite.

Some patients experience muscular pains and aches.

Small gum-boils or blisters may appear in the mouth.

There may be a metallic or unpleasant taste in the mouth for a few hours.

There may be a sensation of burning on the tongue.

There may be a transient reappearance of symptoms of old illnesses.

Some people experience short-lived mood changes.

It is typical for reactions to appear between the second and sixth treatments, although they may be noticed after the assessment, the most common being a sense of relaxation, pleasant tiredness and well-being. The reactions do not generally last longer than twenty-four hours, and although they may be temporarily unpleasant, patients comment at the same time that they are beginning to feel well again.

It is the responsibility of the therapist to distinguish between a reaction and a complication of the illness.

Although the reactions may appear and stay in one system, such as the urinary system, they may also change from treatment to treatment. Their nature and duration are noted on the treatment record at each session.

If the patient experiences very strong reactions, regular warm footbaths should be given, and the patient should have as much rest as possible. If there is any doubt about the reactions, or any question of whether the patient is experiencing a reaction, a side effect of medication or a complication, a doctor must be consulted. Treatment time may also be reduced, or given at less frequent intervals. It must be explained to the patient that such reactions indicate an improvement in the function of the organs concerned, even if the patient does not associate them with the illness. The patient should be reassured that they are only temporary and help towards recovery.

Frequency
of treatment

For the majority of people seeking treatment for conditions such as backache, sinusitis and eczema, twelve treatments, given at twice-weekly intervals will usually be sufficient. Treatment is, however, continued for as long as the patient continues to experience reactions, and only when these have subsided can the series be brought to an end.

Each treatment lasts between twenty and thirty-five minutes, and is followed by a rest period of twenty minutes, or more if necessary, with the patient lying down and undisturbed.

At the first visit, a complete assessment of all the reflex zones of the feet is made. Subsequently, it is explained to the patient that only those areas of the feet which are uncomfortable will be treated. Each disordered reflex zone is treated for up to 20 seconds, less if the patient becomes cold, sweaty, dry-mouthed or hyperventilates before the 20 seconds have passed, when one of the harmonising strokes are used until the patient returns to normal. If possible, all the painful and disordered reflex zones are treated twice during each session and preferably three times. It is, however, the most disordered zones which give rise to coolness and sweating – the 'shock' reactions – so they have to be palpated with care. By treatment is meant probing the area of discomfort or abnormal tissue tonus with the thumb or fingers, releasing the pressure, and again palpating until the discomfort lessens and the tissue tonus becomes more normal.

At the end of the session the patient is left comfortably relaxed, the feet warm and the breathing even, and rests for twenty minutes. If the feet remain cold at the end of the resting period they are warmed with a footbath.

The pattern of treatment changes once the patient begins to experience reactions. Now treatment is first given to the system which is reacting (and this system will often be more sensitive to touch than it was at previous visits), and then to the disordered zones noted on the patient's treatment card. For example, if the patient is being treated for backache, and as a reaction has increased sputum, at the next visit the whole of the respiratory system is treated as well as all other painful and disordered reflex zones. If the reactions change to an increased urinary output at the next visit, the whole of the urinary system and all the other disordered zones are treated.

A treatment card which shows all of the reflex zones is completed after the assessment. Any visual abnormalities are indicated with shading; painful and disordered reflex zones are marked on a scale of one to five; those marked five requiring the most intensive treatment.

As treatment progresses changes occur in the feet. The following are signs of general improvement:

- feet which have been cold become warm;
- feet which were rigid and stiff become more malleable;
- reflex zones which were painful may become more painful initially, but as treatment continues the discomfort on palpation is reduced;
- reactions are not too strong;
- changes in the expression, voice and general bearing of the patient;
- increasing mobility;
- pain and symptoms subside;
- sleep improves and becomes more restful;
- general alertness improves.

It is important that at every treatment those reflex zones which are painful or disordered at the first assessment are treated. When they are no longer painful to normal touch on palpation, and the tissue tonus is again normal, it is no longer necessary to include them in the treatment session.

It may be that at the end of a course of twelve treatments many of the disorders on the feet have disappeared, but some painful reflex zones remain. Once the reactions have ceased the treatment is stopped, but may be resumed in another series at a later stage, after an interval of a few weeks when a new assessment is made.

For someone who is terminally ill or has long-standing chronic illness, treatment which alleviates symptoms may be continued for as long as it is helpful to the patient, and it is only necessary to treat those areas of the feet which relate to the symptoms the patient is experiencing. For example, if the person is constipated, it is generally helpful to treat the whole of the intestinal tract and the solar plexus. If the patient needs help with expectoration, as in children with cystic fibrosis, the whole of the respiratory system is treated, also the solar plexus. If the patient has pain over an operation site or an open wound, then gentle holding of the related area on the feet will often relieve some and sometimes all of the pain. A comment which is often made by such patients is that during therapy they 'feel like a person again, and not like a patient'.

First-aid treatment may be given when an injury has been sustained, or for pain such as earache, or discomfort such as travel sickness. If the injury is to the knee, a firm, sustained hold is maintained over the reflex zone to the knee for two or three minutes, until the pain eases. For travel sickness or nausea, the reflex zone to the solar plexus or the stomach is held on either hands or feet until the sickness passes. For hiccoughs or persistent coughing the reflex zones to the solar plexus and the diaphragm are held for two to three minutes. After an epidural anaesthetic the reflex zones to the back at the level of the injection site are likewise held for two to three minutes.

When the patient is suffering from a chronic degenerative disease such as multiple sclerosis or rheumatoid arthritis, treatment needs to be given over a much longer period. Twice-weekly sessions are given until the reactions begin (which may take longer to appear in people with multiple sclerosis), and may then be spread out over weekly or fortnightly intervals, for as long as there are reactions. If the patient derives mobility, comfort or an improved sense of well-being, it is worthwhile to continue treating them regularly, even if they do not have strong physical reactions. There is ofen improved benefit if there are occasional short breaks in the therapy.

Palliative treatment can be given, where appropriate, to patients who are terminally ill. This is directed at the relief of distressing symptoms such as diarrhoea, coughing, nausea, vomiting, hiccoughs, itching, restlessness and pain. In many such patients there is gross distortion of tissue tonus and sensitivity, and the feet either do not feel any discomfort during therapy, they may be wholly insensitive, or they may be hypersensitive. In such patients frequent soothing, stroking movements and any of the harmonisation holds interspersed between the palpation of treatment help to make the treatment comfortable and relieving.

Healthy reflex zones are not painful to touch. Only when there is some disorder in the part of the body related to that reflex zone does the patient become aware of discomfort. The patient's perception of pain or discomfort or sensation may be altered in the following circumstances:

- when taking drugs, particularly steroids, beta-blockers, pain killers;
- when taking hypnotics, tranquillisers and hormone replacement therapy;
- during chemotherapy and radiotherapy;
- in terminal illness;
- in psychotic conditions;
- in periphero-vascular disease;
- in paralysis;
- in brain tumours or any central nervous system disorders;
- in vitamin deficiency.

Where the findings on the feet do not match the known history of the patient or the observations of the therapist, the conditions listed above should be considered.

OTHER REFLEX ZONES

There are reflex zones on the hands, the back, the neck and the face, and if it is not possible to use the feet because of wounds or amputation, then treatment can be given on any of these surfaces. It is a common finding that people respond more to treatment on the feet and back than on the hands and face except in certain circumstances.

If the reactions are very strong or the feet very painful, therapy can be given to different areas or alternated with therapy to the feet until the patient's condition improves and treatment on the feet becomes more tolerable. Sometimes the therapist will choose another area if the treatment has reached a plateau, in an endeavour to find out which is the best mode of treatment for that patient at that particular time.

The patient may be shown how to hold or rub parts of the hand for first aid relief.

Contra-indications
for treatment

Treatment should only be given where the patient is at ease with the therapy and the therapist. Some people do not like their feet being touched, and some people dislike treatment which involves physical touch, just as others would not choose acupuncture as they dislike the thought of needles puncturing the skin. Seriously ill and dying patients may, on occasions, not want treatment on a given day or at that particular hour. Such feelings must be respected where one is trying to coax the patient into recovery. As with food, treatment given in small doses at frequent intervals serves the needs of such patients best. Do not treat:

* if the patient does not want treatment;
* if the reactions are very strong and affect several systems at the same time;
* if the patient has hyperpyrexia;
* pregnant women in the first trimester if they have a previous history of miscarriage, or if they are threatening to abort;
* when an acute infectious illness is present;
* when there is an acute local infection of the feet, such as cellulitis;
* if the patient has had a deep vein thrombosis in the past six months;
* in acute infections of the lymphatic system;

- when patients feel faint during treatment (this usually happens within a few minutes of the commencement of therapy);
- in epilepsy, unless the practitioner is sufficiently experienced;
- in psychoses;
- when the feet are gangrenous, burned, injured or severely infected;
- when there are any abnormal responses to treatment;
- when the patient needs surgery; for example, in ectopic pregnancy.

Treatment
during pregnancy, labour and the puerperium

Treatment during labour and the puerperium is a special subject outside the scope of this chapter. Only a few general principles will be given.

Reflex zone therapy can be helpful during pregnancy when the pregnancy is normal and when the minor complications of pregnancy arise, but the woman must be under the care of her doctor and the midwife. If there is a specific problem such as backache, the treatment pattern is the same as for any other patient; namely, an assessment is done and then all the painful and disordered reflex zones are treated. If treatment is part of a programme to minimise the problems which may arise, it may be given regularly at more widely spaced intervals. If the woman experiences an improved sense of well-being with treatment, it may be given regularly.

During labour, reflex zone therapy is best carried out by the midwife and is used to relieve backache during the first stage; to sedate labour pains which are too strong when the labour threatens to become precipitate; and to stimulate contractions which become too weak or too irregular. If a third person is present and is giving therapy, that person always acts under the instructions of the midwife.

During the third stage, treatment may be given by an experienced midwife to assist in the delivery of the placenta, especially when it is slow to separate.

During the puerperium, treatment is relaxing for most women, and can help with pain in the perineum following episiotomy, backache, and in both helping the milk flow to get started and to keep it flowing, as well as with sleep and the pains of involution. Only a qualified midwife may attend a mother and baby during labour and for ten days after birth. Reflex zone therapy may be given by someone who is not a midwife, and at the request of the mother, but the therapist must always act under the instruction of the midwife.

Some midwives report that treatment is helpful in assisting conception when failure to conceive is due to tension. At the same time the customary advice is given on technique, fertile times for conception, and nutrition.

Treatment used by midwives is a separate, specialised field. The process is a normal one, but mother and baby are involved, complications may arise, and when they do they usually arise quickly and may be life-threatening. Only experienced midwives and those practised in therapy should treat women with any complication of pregnancy, particularly hyperemesis gravidarum and pre-eclamptic toxaemia. Reflex zone therapy is absolutely contra-indicated in women with placenta praevia.

Babies and small children usually respond well to treatment, and incubator babies are now known to need the stimulus of touch. There are several reports of such babies becoming calmer with treatment on the feet and effleurage.

Scars

After surgery or trauma, areas of the feet corresponding to parts of the body where recent or past surgery or trauma have occurred are found to be painful on palpation. Tonsils are a common example. There are special techniques for treating such areas, but they are always included in therapy at each session until they become less painful. One method is for the therapist to lightly cross-hatch the area with a fingernail, and then apply gentle pressure to the whole area until the discomfort ceases.

After surgery – for example, cholecystectomy – the area on the dorsum of the right foot which corresponds to the operation site and the solar plexus are held for two or three minutes in a light but firm manner. This often enhances the effect of pain-relieving drugs.

The versatility of this simple form of treatment enables it to be adapted to many situations. In practised and skilled hands it offers patients a sense of relaxation and well-being, pain relief, and a form of treatment which may reduce to a greater or lesser extent the need for medicines.

References

1 W.H. Fitzgerald and E.F. Bowers, **Zone Therapy**, *Columbus, Ohio: I.W. Long*, 1917.

2 Chartered Society of Physiotherapy, **Scope of Practice**, Rule 1.

3 A. Lafuente, M. Noguera, C. Puy, A. Molins, F. Titus and F. Sanz, Effekt der Reflexonbehandlung am Fuss bezüglich der prophylaktischen Behandlung mit Flunarazin bei an Cephalea-Kopfschmerzen leidenden Patienten, **Erfahrungsheilkunde** 11: 713–15, 1990.

Further Reading

S. Baldwin **Complementary health**, *Nursing*, 4(46): 15–17, 1991.

A. Lett, **Putting their best feet forward**, *Nursing Times*, 79(34): 49–51, 1983.

H. Marquardt, **Reflex Zone Therapy of the Feet**, *Wellingborough: Thorsons*, 1984.

K. May, **'A new venture in health care'**, *Health Visitor*, 62: 211–13, July 1989.

H. Passant, M. Evans and M. Smith, **Complementary therapies in nursing practice**, *Nursing Times*, 86(4): 25–32, 1990.

D. Rankin-Box, **Complementary therapies in nursing**, *Nursing*, 4(46): 12–14, 1991.

D. Rankin-Box (ed.), **Complementary Health Therapies, A Guide for Nurses and the Caring Professions**, *London: Croom Helm*, 1988.

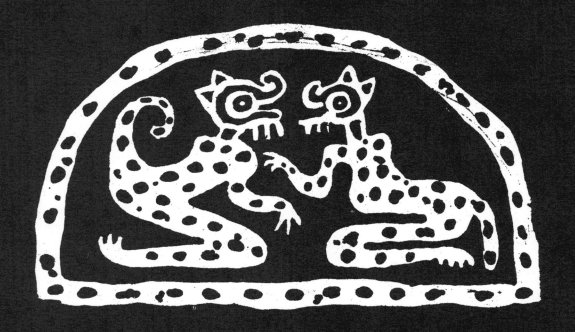

10

HUMOUR THERAPY

Jane Mallett

I made the joyous discovery that 10 minutes of genuine belly laughter had an anaesthetic effect and would give me at least two hours of pain-free sleep. When the painkilling effect of the laughter wore off, we would switch on the motion-picture projector again, and, not infrequently, it would lead to another pain-free sleep interval.[1]

Most humour, laughter and smiling therapy and research into them appears to emanate from the United States. Since evidence suggests that the use of humour, laughter and smiling is related to culture it is difficult to write knowledgeably about the impact of such therapies within the United Kingdom. In addition, a considerable proportion of the research is conducted on healthy adults and is non-clinical in origin. This has resulted in a lack of formal and rigorous evaluation of humour, laughter and smiling therapies. Research, theory, and other literature from a variety of sources have therefore been chosen to discuss the psychological, social and physiological uses and effects of humour, laughter and smiling and their *potential* as therapeutic tools within the UK clinical environment. This approach inevitably makes this chapter slightly different from others in this book.

Definitions
of humour, laughter and smiling

HUMOUR

Humour can be viewed from many different frameworks, and has been studied from the positions of sociology, physiology and psychology. The many perspectives in which humour can be perceived may account for the difficulty in defining humour. In a social sense, this is illustrated by Moody,[2] who describes no less than six ways in which a person may be thought to have a 'good sense of humour' – that is, a person who laughs easily at another's jokes; a person who laughs at jokes that others appreciate; a person who is the 'life and soul of the party'; a person who produces new, original, humorous remarks; a person who can laugh at himself or herself; and a person who sees the 'funny side of life'.

The things that we respond to as humorous employ a multitude of often subtle techniques to create the humour, which Berger[3] has grouped into four categories: the use of language (for example, irony or puns); the use of logic (such as analogy or absurdity); the use of identity (for instance, caricature or imitation); and the use of action (like slapstick or chase scenes).

LAUGHTER

Laughter, on the other hand, is *usually* taken to be the physical manifestation of humour or joy. Gelotology, or the science of laughter, thus refers to events occurring in association with humorous experiences – namely, the stimulus of humour, the emotional response or 'mirth' and the accompanying behaviour, such as laughter or giggling.[4]

However, although laughter can be described adequately in physical terms, to assume that it is merely the expression of appreciated humour or joy would be too simplistic because laughter is also socially organised with talk and body movement, and is used by participants in meaningful ways, which will be discussed later.

SMILING

Smiling has also been described in physical terms by Chapman[5] as 'an upward stretching of the mouth occurring without vocal sound but possibly accompanied by loud exhalations of breath, particularly at its inception'. Whilst smiling can be related to humour and laughter, it may also be used on its own in a social context as an appeasing device.[6] Furthermore, it may reflect intimate or affiliative behaviour,[7] and may have originated from a display of submission.[8]

This chapter will attempt to illustrate the psychological, social and physical effects and uses of humour, laughter and smiling, how they are used naturally by patients and health-care professionals, and the potential benefits that may arise. In addition, the advantages and disadvantages of humour therapy, based on evidence from research and individual case histories, will be discussed.

The historical
context

People have written about humour from the time of the Greek philosophers onwards. Plato and his pupil Aristotle were amongst the earliest writers reflecting the 'superiority theory' of humour.[9] The Bible tells us of the positive benefit of humour: 'A cheerful heart does good like a medicine: but a broken spirit makes one sick' (Proverbs 17:22).[10]

Goldstein[11] and Moody[2] review the ways in which humour has been perceived, and also reveal an interesting account of the history of laughter as a therapeutic tool. For example, the thirteenth-century surgeon Henri de Mondeville suggested that laughter may aid post-operative recovery; whilst Gottlieb Hufeland, a nineteenth-century German professor, thought that laughter was an important aid to digestion. In the sixteenth century it was believed that 'mirth' was a cure for melancholy, and that laughter was healthy because it was a form of physical exercise. The seventeenth-century sociologist Herbert Spencer thought that laughter helped release tension, whilst Immannual Kant, the eighteenth-century German philosopher, wrote that laughter promoted the restoration of equilibrium and thus has a favourable influence on health.

Goldstein was of the opinion, however, that despite the extolling of medical benefits, the moral view of laughter was generally negative in England, and that it has only been within the last century that laughter in public has been socially acceptable. With perception he writes:

> Victorian England, not surprisingly, frowned on laughter. . . . While girls and women were permitted to smile in deference or to giggle at the slightest suggestion of impropriety, they were not allowed to laugh with glee. They could be embarrassed but not happy. (Today, of course, they may be happy, but not embarrassed.)[11]

Thus, since the time of Plato, various aspects of humour and laughter have been studied and many theories developed. The theories often reflect different outlooks and ideological perspectives, and as such demonstrate the many facets and holistic nature of humour. Bellert indicates that humour theory evolved in three phases (see Table 10.1).[12] Although the whole story is probably more complex than this, it does give an idea of the changes in opinions over the last few thousand years. The term 'theory' is loosely applied here since it refers only to the concepts that authors have put forward, which in some cases are descriptions of conditions under which humour may be experienced rather than an attempt to explain humour.[13]

Other humour theories which do not appear to be classified by Bellert[12] or are categorised in different ways are listed below. For example, although Bellert places Spencer and Darwin in a pre-theoretical category, it is arguable that they are presenting a biological, instinct or evolutionary theory.

Table 10.1 Three phases of humour theory development

Theory	Author	Date	Further comments
Pre-theoretical	Plato, Aristotle		
	Proverbs		Biblical writings
	Joubert	1560	`Body fluids'
	Hobbes	1651	Superiority
	Kant	1790	Incongruity
	Spencer	1860	Tension relief
	Darwin	1890	Comparison between expressions of humans and apes; laughter as a social communication in early infancy
	Sully	1902	Social pleasure
Psychoanalytic	Freud	1905	Psychoanalysis
	McDougall	1903	Laughter as a pain antidote
	Piddington	1933	Compensatory theory
	Eastman	1936	Pleasurable expression
	Fry	1963	Metacommunication and paradox in humour
Cognitive	Koestler	1964	Bisociation (incompatible cognition)
	Berlyne	1972	Arousal jag
	Berger	1976	Bipolar opposition: incongruity
	Leventhal and Cupchik	1976	Humour judgement model
	Wilson	1979	Social-cognitive conservative
	Morreaull	1983	Pleasant psychological shift
	Kuhlman	1984	Humour stimulus–response model
	Ziv	1984	Cognitive process of local logic
	Lefcourt and Martin	1986	Humour and life stress
	Apte	1988	Humourology: conceptualisation

Source: J.L. Bellert, (1989) `Humor: A Therapeutic Approach in Oncology Nursing', *Cancer Nursing*, 12(2): 65–70, Table 1. Three Phases of Humor Theory Development.[12]

Surprise theories: E.g., Darwin,[14] Descartes,[15] and Hobbes;[16] *Ambivalence theories*: E.g. Descartes[15] and Joubert;[17] *Configurational theories*; *Conflict theories*; *Dualist theories*; *Gestalt theories*; *Piagetian theories*; *Mastery theories*: see Keith-Spiegel,[13] Robinson[9] and Wilson.[18]

SUMMARY

Many have described the numerous uses and effects of humour, laughter and smiling, and many varied theories are used to categorise and illustrate them, some of which have been mentioned above. Perhaps because humour can be used in a multiplicity of ways and has diverse effects, it is particularly difficult to define, or to explain adequately or understand from one viewpoint or theory alone all the activities and meanings that are inherent in a humorous interaction.

Use
of humour in society

In 1952, Radcliffe-Brown[19] published his now famous work *Structure and Function in Primitive Society*. In this he distinguished between symmetrical joking relationships, where each party has the right to tease, and asymmetrical relationships where only one party is so privileged.[20] He defined the joking relationship as a 'relation between two persons in which one is by custom permitted, and, in some instances required, to tease or make fun of the other, who in turn is required to take no offense'[19]

Studies of African societies have indicated that the so-called 'joking relationship' is not developed amongst the Swazi,[21] and the nearest approach to a joking relationship in the Ashanti is a privileged familiarity.[22] However, it is present among the Lozi of Northern Rhodesia[23] and prevails symmetrically among cross-cousins of the Tswana where it is reported by some informants to make for tolerance and indulgence between husband and wife – thus ensuring a stable marriage.[24] Other informants, however, maintain that the joking relationship has the opposite effect, since a wife may be cheeky and impertinent to her husband and not show him the deference and submission due to him.[24]

Humour can be used in contrasting or similar ways in different societies. For example, humour has been reported to be used by Greenland Eskimos to resolve their quarrels. Each is said to produce humorous insults and obscene jokes ridiculing the opponent: the one who induces most laughter from the audience wins.[9] Eskimos are also reported to use ridicule against thievery, laughing whenever the thief's name is mentioned and that – perhaps consequently – stealing is almost unknown among the Eskimos.[25]

Instances of humour being used trans-culturally are those of 'gallows humour' and 'ethnic humour'. According to Robinson,[9] gallows humour appears to be produced in dangerous situations, or as a 'macabre humour' where bravado is shown in the face of death'. Obrdlik,[25] on the basis of his experiences in Czechoslovakia following the advent of Hitler, describes the positive effect of gallows humour in the strengthening of morale among oppressed people, and the negative effect upon those towards whom it is directed. He also felt that the social influence of gallows humour was enormous, and quotes this example:

> To find a Czech who is truly loyal to the Germans is no easy task. According to Czech gallows humor, the Gestapo found one such specimen at long last. He was an old man walking up and down the street and speaking seriously to himself aloud: 'Adolf Hitler is the greatest leader. The Germans are a noble nation. I would rather work for ten Germans than for one Czech.' When the Gestapo agent asked what was his occupation, the Czech admirer of nazism reluctantly confessed that he was a gravedigger.

This type of humour was also used by the Americans in World War II and the Vietnam War.[9]

Ethnic jokes use the stereotypes, personality traits or the conflicts of particular groups. Comedians and analysts claim that humour is the primary factor in changing the status of minority groups and in reducing racial prejudice.[9] This is partially supported by LaFave and Mannell,[26] who argue that ethnic humour can be used to furnish positive information about an ethnic group, and to alert people to cultural relativity, and could diminish ethnocentric bigotry and feelings of superiority. They conclude that a surprising amount of evidence exists for the humanitarian functions of humour. Others however, would argue strongly against this view, believing instead that such 'humour' reinforces stereotypical images.[27]

Opinions remain divided, and a joke may cause both offence and agreement. A recent example was provided by a quip from comedian Jim Davidson, suggesting that women could not drive or fly planes because they suffered from premenstrual tension. Thames TV reportedly received complaints from 'outraged' viewers and was reprimanded by the Broadcasting Standards Council. However, the National Association for Premenstrual Syndrome considered asking Jim Davidson to become their patron for, as the secretary of the organisation stated, 'occasionally he gets it right'.[27]

Use
of humour and laughter
in Western health care

It appears that so far most humour and laughter therapy and research is confined to the United States, and that most humour advocates practise in the medical, nursing or psychotherapy professions. There is also some support from patients who have experienced the use of humour and laughter in the clinical environment.[28,29] While individual case histories and small quasi-experimental studies from many sources provide a great deal of support for humour and laughter therapy, and when it is, or is not, appropriate to utilise this[2,30–38] it would seem a pertinent time to conduct larger, formal and perhaps multicentred studies to evaluate immediate and long-term physical, psychological and social outcomes. Although humour therapy appears to produce positive results, further research is required to give a more detailed picture of how, why, for whom and when.

Effects
and uses of humour, laughter and smiling

Humour, laughter and smiling have a number of effects and uses which have been divided into psychological, social and physical aspects. All these effects may, of course, appear simultaneously and may have been encouraged or utilised by participants in order to do this. For example, in social interaction, humour could be used to 'smooth the way'.

PSYCHOLOGICAL EFFECTS AND USES OF HUMOUR

Humour has been demonstrated to have beneficial psychological outcomes. This relates to its role as a stress-buffer,[39] a coping mechanism[30,40–42] and its potential ability to reduce anxiety and stress levels.[43–45] The developmental stages of humour with increasing age have also been studied.[46] Humour also has a moderating effect on the relation between negative life events and mood disturbance. People who score low on humour measures have higher correlations between negative life events and mood disturbance than subjects with high humour scores. This lends support to the notion of humour as a stress-buffer. This is because humorists can distance themselves from the immediate threat of a predicament and view it from a different perspective.[39] The results of three related studies concluded that there was considerable support for the hypotheses that humour reduces the impact of stress. However, in order for the humour to be utilised in this way, the individual must place a high value on humour and make use of this in stressful situations.

Differences have been found in humour utilisation and appreciation between males and females.[47,48] As stress and psychological distress increases, females tend to see the humorous side of things, whereas no correlation was found for males.[42] The latter study also indicated that humour does not moderate the effect of life stress, but may be of use in coping with some situations.

It is possible that humour also has a part in reducing anxiety levels. In a study by Nemeth,[45] people shown a humorous film had significantly decreased anxiety levels, while groups shown a non-humorous film did not. Although there were some concerns regarding variables within the research, it was felt that there was a direct relationship between humour and anxiety.

A study of twenty-four people over sixty-five years of age found significant positive relationships between situational humour and perceived health, situational humour and morale, and a significant negative relationship between coping humour and perceived health. Therefore, people with a higher level of situational humour had a greater perceived health status and morale than those with lower levels, and the greater the use of coping humour, the lower was a person's perceived health.[49]

Humour which appears to demonstrate conflict, such as that about sexuality and the elderly, can be used to communicate about emotional and psychological issues.[50] As an example,

> In preparation for his marriage to a girl many years his junior, a gay old dog went to his doctor for advice as to how he could keep his bride satisfied. The doctor took one look at the withered old fellow, shook his head, and said, 'I think the best thing for you to do is take in a young boarder.' Several months after the wedding, the old man dropped in for a check-up and proudly announced that his new wife was pregnant. The doctor winked, and said, 'I guess you took my advice about that boarder.' 'Sure did. And she's pregnant too'[50]

It is likely that therapists and health-care professionals have shown interest in the use of humour because of its potential stress-buffering, anxiety-reducing roles and use in communication. There is now a growing field of research within these areas which indicates that this might be so.[12]

SOCIAL EFFECTS AND USES OF HUMOUR

Humour can be viewed as an interpersonal asset or liability depending on the perceptions that others have of the person producing the humour. Mettee *et al.*[51] found in a quasi-experiment using students that a demonstration of a sense of humour by 'potential' lecturers could elicit negative or positive responses from an audience dependent on the reputation of the lecturer. Successful humour was found to increase perceived competence of 'aloof' potential lecturers, whereas it did not change the perceived competence of 'clownish' potential lecturers.

Studies have also shown that social variables affect humour appreciation, and the majority of sociologists agree that jokes only become jokes as a result of the social responses to them.[52] It was found that male students, where possible, would use humour appreciation of sexual humour as a means of communicating interest in the (attractive) female experimenter.[53] In addition, Martineau's model of the social functions of humour suggest that humour directed towards a group will have different effects subject to whether the humour is initiated within or from the outside group, and whether the humour is disparaging or enhances the in-group's or out-group's esteem.[54] This relates to La Fave and Mannell's study [26] of ethnic humour which suggests that both positive and negative effects may result from this type of humour.

There is also evidence to suggest that sick joke cycles can be a form of 'collective mental hygienic defense mechanism' which allows people in society to articulate and cope with the worst disasters.[55] For example, this joke followed President John F. Kennedy's assassination in 1963: 'What were JFK's last words upon leaving Washington, DC?' 'I need a trip to Dallas like a hole in the head'. Or after the Challenger explosion in 1986: 'Where do astronauts go on vacation? All over Florida'. And after the Chernobyl disaster, also in 1986: 'What's the weather in Kiev? Overcast and 10,000 degrees'.

SOCIAL EFFECTS AND USES OF LAUGHTER

From a sociological viewpoint, Jefferson *et al.* define laughter as 'systematically produced, socially organised activity'.[56] Laughter as a social experience was demonstrated in a series of experiments by Chapman.[5] The results showed that a companion's presence and responsiveness affected the laughter and smiling of others. This influence depended on the amount the companion smiled, looked at the other's face, how closely they sat together and their body orientation, and whether or not the companion encroached on the other's 'space' when laughing. It was concluded that 'The mere addition of a second companion is not sufficient to enhance laughter and smiling, but the degree to which two companions look at one another can be an important determinant of responsiveness to humour.'

This is supported by other research in a restaurant, which indicates that people who were alone laughed less.[7] A sex and age difference also occurred, where adult females were observed to laugh more frequently than males. Among females, the younger age group of twelve to seventeen years laughed most compared to males, where the eighteen to twenty-two years age group laughed most frequently. These studies support the theory that laughter is not just a physical response to humour but is also related to the social activity and environment.

Humour and laughing are invitations which aim at reducing social distance and those who do not laugh while others are laughing can be defined as 'bad sports'.[57] The view of laughter as an invitation to which one participant may invite another is also reiterated by Jefferson.[58] The only time that laughter or a joke is produced and a serious response is expected is when the joker is 'troubles-telling'; for example, when a person makes a joke and/or laughs while conveying a trouble, the hearer is expected to take the trouble seriously and not to laugh.

SOCIAL EFFECTS AND USES OF SMILING

Smiling, like laughter, appears to be used in a social context. It may be utilised to indicate a willingness to engage in social interaction and a posture of friendliness and non-hostility.[6,59] In addition, smiling is more frequent in females than males and is thought to be consistent with the notion that females exhibit more affiliative and intimate behaviour and have a less aggressive role.[6,7]

PHYSICAL EFFECTS AND USES OF HUMOUR AND LAUGHTER

The physiological effects of humour and laughter have also been extensively researched. A study by Godkewitsch [60], for example, has shown that heart rate, basal skin resistance and galvanic skin response are related to joke-bodies (that is, the main or middle part of the joke) and punchlines. It was also noted that physiological responses to punchlines were associated with their funniness in the predicted direction. That is, in general, the more arousal evoked, the funnier the jokes were rated.[60,61]

A review of the literature by Fry[4] indicated that laughing affects most of the major systems in our bodies. He also indicated that heart rate is positively correlated with laughing. This produces an increase in blood pressure, reflects stimulation of heart muscle activity and may be due to the resultant increased abdominal pressure and venous return following the activation of the respiratory system. This may be of benefit to patients who have suffered from myocardial infarction, where regular exercise has been found to aid recovery. Heart rate was found to decrease following laughter, while arterial blood pressure decreased below resting levels.[4,62] It was proposed that this phenomenon contributes to survival by its enhancement of the circulatory system. The musculature system is also affected, in that muscle tone decreases and relaxes in the muscles not used in laughing. There is a positive association between subjective evaluation of a joke's funniness and muscle tension; also, muscle tension decreases post-laughter.[4,5,63] This could be helpful to the patient, and help to terminate the spasm-pain-spasm-pain cycle.[4] The clinical significance of these physiological effects, however, has yet to be evaluated.

The findings of Dillon and colleagues [64] suggest that positive emotional states may enhance the immune system. Salivary immunoglobulin A (IgA) concentration was found to increase significantly after subjects viewed a humorous videotape, compared to no change in immunoglobulin status after a non-humorous videotape was viewed. This study also showed that scores on a 'Coping Humour Questionnaire' were correlated with IgA concentrations prior to viewing either tape. However, there was a negative relationship between the questionnaire scores and difference in IgA concentration before and after viewing the humorous tape. It was inferred that there may be a ceiling to changes in IgA concentrations, and that participants who use humour more often as a coping device are close to that ceiling and therefore will have less increase in IgA concentrations.

Other experimental research also supports the positive effect of humour on the immune system in healthy volunteers. In two studies, one group of five subjects watched a 60-minute humour video (experimental group) while five did not.[65,66] In the first project, the release of plasma adrenalin, cortisol and noradrenaline were measured at time intervals coinciding with before, during and after the video. It was found that those who watched the humorous video had lower adrenalin and cortisol levels. Noradrenaline levels were unchanged. This suggested that mirth can modulate adrenocorticomedullary and possibly immunological activity by suppressing the release of cortisol and adrenalin.[65]

The second experiment by the researchers was set up in a similar manner; this time, however, plasma cortisol and proliferation of lymphocytes were measured to indicate immune activity. It was found that cortisol was decreased significantly in those subjects who had seen the video and spontaneous lymphocyte blastogenesis was significantly increased from baseline. It was concluded that 'humour associated laughter may act as an immunomodulator'.[66]

Another effect of laughter is its ability to increase discomfort thresholds in experimental subjects. The data from the study of Cogan and colleagues[67] also indicated that this was due to the humorous nature of the material rather than the degree of interest of the material alone. It was concluded that laughter may be useful as an intervention for the reduction of pain. Further research is necessary to indicate the value of laughter therapy to patients experiencing pain. All of the above findings may have significant implications for disease *if* they are transferable to the clinical situation.

Natural
uses of humour and laughter by the patient and health-care professionals

The use of humour as a resource to both health-care professionals and patients has been known for over thirty years. Analysis of three months' observation by patients in hospital by Coser[57] suggested that laughter and jocular talk could be understood by: anxiety about self, submission to a rigid authority structure and adjustment to a rigid routine. This type of humour could be used to ward off danger, as a means of rebellion against authority and as a relief from mechanical routine. Humour can also be used by the patients to impart more serious covert messages. Emerson's work[68] showed that . . . 'where staff and patients take for granted that matters related to death, staff competence, and indignities to patients will be discussed circumspectly or avoided, making joking references to these topics are found'. The reason for this appeared to be that a taboo topic can be introduced in joke form, thus suspending a serious framework. The joker (for example the patient) can therefore express potentially risky messages in a covert way. The recipient (for instance the nurse) can either maintain the joke framework or transpose the topic from humorous to serious, thereby inadvertently acknowledging the taboo subject. The joker can either accept the transition or further negotiate to have his or her remarks taken as humorous. The importance of this in a professional–client relationship is that anxious patients who wish to talk about taboo subjects, such as their death, may attempt to introduce them covertly in a humorous framework. It then requires a sensitive health-care professional to pick up these cues and make the decision as to whether the patient does want to continue in a joke framework, in which case by transposing the conversation to a serious framework they are acknowledging the taboo topic themselves. Otherwise, understanding that patients do want to discuss their worries, the professional may reply in a serious context and so give them the opportunity for doing so.

Patients have been found to use humour to convey in an indirect manner feelings such as anxiety, fear, anger, frustration, embarrassment, concern, hope and joy.[30,69] Humour is perceived as being useful in nursing situations to facilitate learning; to alleviate fear, shame, embarrassment, anxiety, stress and tension; to break the ice; to establish warm interpersonal relationships; to dissipate anger, hostility and aggression in a socially acceptable way; to encourage a sense of trust; to lighten the heaviness associated with physical damage and death; to provide an escape from reality; and to circumvent feelings that are too difficult to deal with. In relation to these latter points, the most important concern is that humour should be used for the patient's needs and not to reinforce the pathological denial of reality.[9,70] This is illustrated by the tendency of suicidal patients to tell significantly more jokes with a self-punishing theme than non-suicidal controls.[71]

A study of twelve female and eight male cataract patients, aged sixty-five to ninety-five, indicated that there was a positive relationship between the recovery rate and humour scores of joke rating for the males. Those who scored highest recovered fastest. Although these findings were not significant, they may indicate a trend that requires further investigation.[30] Since it is the nurse's role to help the patient regain and maintain independence in daily living, humour is a vital component of patient-centred, holistic nursing care.[30]

Patients also describe how humour can be used. One such account has been Bruning[28] who, at the age of thirty-one discovered that she had breast cancer. The day following diagnosis she had to have a modified radical mastectomy and later went on to have a course of chemotherapy. She wrote that laughter was one of the best coping mechanisms. To quote from her book:

> There's nothing funny about having cancer, but we can still laugh at the world. Sometimes we can even laugh at ourselves – or appreciate the absurdities involved with our disease and our treatment. It's

hard to imagine laughing when you've been throwing up for three hours straight, and you know you'll be doing the same thing every two weeks for the next year; when you're so weak you can barely drag yourself out of bed; when you're so pale and bald that even you don't want to be seen with you. And yet patients do find it within themselves to laugh. These things are so awful that people need to laugh – as an escape, a defense, and as a release of tension. Patients often joke about looking like Kojak, or majoring in Advanced Toilet Bowl, or how they might get arrested because their arms look like a junkie's. As one patient says, 'It doesn't seem too awful when you laugh about it.'

Cousins' case[1] (see page 214) was probably most instrumental in raising the debate of the therapeutic effect of humour and laughter. In 1964 he had ankylosing spondylitis. Cousins devised his own humour and laughter therapy, which he thought helped him to recover. The fact that this might have been related to a placebo effect did not concern him, as this demonstrated to him the power of the mind in relieving illness.

The use of laughter was shown more generally in a survey of patients in a rehabilitation hospital, which showed that patients welcome laughter and perceive nurses who laugh with their patients to be therapeutic.[38] Further research by Van Zandt and LaFont[72] demonstrates that professionals consciously and subconsciously use humour. A questionnaire sent to nurses to ascertain if there is therapeutic value in humour suggested that it was used consciously to help the patients cope, to reduce their anxiety and stress, and also as a communication tool.

Health-care professionals also utilise humour to help themselves. Professionals who are constantly faced with patients' deaths learn to make use of 'black humour'. Although this may seem to indicate lack of feeling, it generally demonstrates the opposite.[73] This is supported by Coombs and Goldman's observational study[40] over three months, of an intensive care unit which showed that one of the most common techniques to manage emotional stress by professionals was the use of humour. It was found that much joking and kidding occurred almost every night and that patients were also sometimes drawn into the joking. It was also felt that the staff's lightheartedness in the midst of such painful human drama would seem inappropriate to most observers, but they felt that rather than interfere with the staff's ability to do a good job it actually contributed to the quality of their performance.

Humour is not, however, a universal panacea. If tension or stress levels are too high humour will fall 'flat' or become ineffective.[40,70,74] Humour must obviously be used at the right time, in the right situation and in the right amount.[9]

Applications
and potential benefits of humour and laughter therapy

Because of the psychological, social and physical effects and uses of humour, laughter and smiling, there are a number of ways in which they can be useful in therapy. It is likely that health-care professionals can greatly influence humour, laughter and smiling in patients and hence its effect on their physical well-being and the building of the therapeutic situation. A consideration for health-care professionals is that the degree of social intimacy is a crucial factor influencing 'humorous laughter'[5] and that smiling may be used to demonstrate friendliness and non-hostility[6,59] and could possibly be used to promote this.

Humour therapy is utilised by nurses in various ways: to take people's mind off pain, to relax patients, to make patients 'feel good', as part of 'humour reminiscence' with dying patients, or as a tool for interpersonal communication.[12,75] Also of relevance for health care and professional–client relationships is that affiliation occurs when laughing together, and that ongoing laughter can be renewed and extended. Of especially strong affiliative importance could be laughing together, not just at the same moment but also in the same manner.[56]

It has been reported that clowns and clowning can be used successfully in humour therapy. Psychiatric patients who were exposed to a clown troupe demonstrated increased social interaction the following day. Patients who previously did not talk began to discuss the clowns' visit with other patients.[32] Adults and children alike are said to react to clowns. One famous clown who, when walking through a hospital, saw a child with a doll like himself, went over to the child, who spoke his name. The child had been unresponsive for over six months and was diagnosed as catatonic.[2] In another case history a clown visited a ninety-five-year-old man with severe depression who had not eaten or spoken for several days. His doctors were concerned that he was soon going to die. Within 30 minutes the man was talking, laughing and eating, and lived for several more years, maintaining communication with the clown.[2]

Humour also has a role in teaching:

> The use of humor during the teaching process is also helpful in allaying tensions and fears surrounding the learning experience. Humor permits individuals to ask questions they may otherwise not ask, and to hear instructions they may otherwise be too anxious to hear. A humorous joke or comment can break through resistance to learning.[12]

Other research has provided data for the importance of humour and laughter therapy. The development and evaluation of a programme of 'humorous activities' on the well-being of senior adults found that mood levels were significantly elevated by humorous activity and that there was a transitory enhancement of subjective well-being, although there was no evidence that this had a lasting effect.[35]

Laughter has also been successfully used as a therapy facilitator with adult aphasics.[37] Two female subjects of eighty-four and seventy-nine years who had incurred cerebrovascular accidents (with mild-to-moderate expressive language deficit characterised by word-finding difficulties and high-level language formulation difficulties, and severe receptive and expressive language impairments characterised by auditory comprehension and memory deficits respectively) listened to a laughter tape in between their therapy tasks. The results indicated that both women made substantial gains over the baseline when humour/laughter was introduced into therapy. However, when the laughter tape was withdrawn, the target behaviours decelerated towards the baseline. Qualitative differences were also noted in that humour or laughter provided an excellent 'ice-breaker'. The authors supported the use of humour and laughter intervention but felt that more precise research should be undertaken to evaluate their effects as positive reinforcers of motivational devices.[37]

Other researchers suggest that 'negatively' toned humour can establish rapport. A study of the therapeutic relationship between health-care professional and client indicated that the topic of humour was mostly related to the client's and therapist's concerns, but that a large percentage of the humorous remarks demonstrated an intense and intimate relationship between the two. It was concluded that humour can be used therapeutically but that successful humour is contextual and spontaneous and that it should be allowed to emerge naturally.[33] Therefore the nature and purpose (and understanding) of humour will depend on the situation.

Potential
disadvantages of humour and laughter therapy

Whether or not to use humour or laughter therapy needs careful consideration. Many of those writing about these types of therapy are very enthusiastic regarding their benefits. Warnings about its appropriateness are less evident, although some authors do provide a more balanced view and it appears to be generally agreed that humour is best used with caution.[74,76,77]

The type of humour utilised in psychotherapy should be precisely appraised. Therapy should not include 'kidding' the clients merely to evoke laughter, since this could lead to the possibility of a therapy session degenerating into 'cheap wisecrack'.[41] Humour can also be detrimental where there exists a lack of mutual respect, and growth-retarding if it becomes a substitute for required change.[78]

Not many authors are as extreme as Kubie[31], who goes as far as to suggest that humour has a very limited role in psychotherapy. He believes that the use of humour by the psychiatrist is potentially destructive (although not always so), and comments that,

> Over the [patient's] desperation the therapist's humor runs a steamroller. I have picked up traces of patients' delayed, bitter responses to the lighthearted or bantering approach of the therapist more often than I care to contemplate.

In addition, negative or snide humour can bring people 'down', and since some state that it cannot be seen as therapeutic it has no place in health care.[75] However, opinions differ on this.[33] The discrepancy may result from lack of agreement on what constitutes negative humour.

Even the best-intentioned humour can have detrimental effects. A case from personal experience illustrates this. A male patient, known for his sense of humour and who had a joking relationship with many nurses, was teased pre-operatively about the discomfort associated with his coming cholecystectomy. His response was always to laugh and joke back. After his operation he confided that he was really worried at the amount of pain that he would have after his operation. This was a situation in which humour had been used with good intent but without sensitivity, since it had obviously caused the patient distress.

Summary

The study of humour, laughter and smiling indicates that these activities could have beneficial psychological, social and physiological effects for clients and health-care professionals. Humour is likely to remove, or help the patient to cope with, many of the problems and anxieties that illness or hospitalisation might cause. It can be used to encourage patients to talk and respond with others and improve their mood. In addition, some have suggested that humour has a particular role to play in patient education. This may be related to the recognition of the importance of counselling, reduction of anxiety and appreciation of the patients' education needs from their perspective, as well as the more obvious process of information-giving, as being necessary for effective health-care teaching.

Laughter may help to improve physical well-being because of the exercise and relaxation it provides, as well as its possible advantage as an analgesic. The affiliative potential of laughter and smiling has relevance for the treatment of clients as well as the development of the therapeutic relationship on which so much depends. Humour and laughter have also been related to positive changes in the immune system.

However, the role of professionals in relation to humour, laughter and smiling must be based on sensitivity and understanding to ensure that the effects on their clients are therapeutic and not destructive. In addition, there is a need for assessment of the effects on patients in the clinical field rather than on healthy individuals, for although humour, laughter and smiling appear therapeutic, there is little empirical evidence to support their effect on clinical outcome.

In a few words:

- Humour, laughter and smiling produce psychological, social and physiological effects; some of these may be beneficial.
- Humour, laughter and smiling may be useful therapeutically.
- Humour and laughter are not always appropriate; use carefully.
- Further research is necessary in order to define effects.

References

1   N. Cousins, Anatomy of an illness (as perceived by the patient), **New England Journal of Medicine**, 295(26): 1458–63, 1976.

2   R.A. Moody, **Laugh after Laugh. The Healing Power of Humor**, Jacksonville. Florida: Headwaters Press, 1978.

3   A.A. Berger, Anatomy of the joke, **Journal of Communication**, 26: 113–15, 1976.

4   W.F. Fry, Humor, physiology, and the aging process, Chapter 4, pp. 81–98, In: L. Nahemow, K.A. McCluskey-Fawcett and P.E. McGhee (eds), **Humor and Aging**, London: Academic Press, 1986.

5   A.J. Chapman, Social aspects of humourous laughter, Chapter 8, pp. 155–85, In: A.J. Chapman and H.C. Foot, **Humor and Laughter: Theory, Research and Applications**, London: John Wiley and Sons, 1976.

6   W.C. Mackey, Parameters of the smile as a social system, **The Journal of Genetic Psychology**, 129: 125–30, 1976.

7   R.M. Adams and B. Kirkevold, Looking, smiling, laughing and moving in restaurants: sex and age differences, **Environmental Psychology and Non-Verbal Behavior**, 3(2): 117–21, 1978.

8   J.S. Lockhard, C.E. Fahrenbruch, J.L. Smith, and C.J. Morgan, Smiling and laughter. Different phyletic origins? **Bulletin of the Psychonomic Society**, 10(3): 183–6, 1977.

9   V.R. Robinson, **Humor and the Health Professions**, USA: Charles B. Slack, Inc, 1977.

10 **The Living Bible**, Great Britain: Tyndale House Publishers, 1971.

11 J.H. Goldstein, A laugh a day. Can mirth keep disease at bay? **Science**, 22: 21–5, 1982.

12 J.L. Bellert, Humor, a therapeutic approach in oncology nursing, **Cancer Nursing**, 12(2): 65–70, 1989.

13 P. Keith-Spiegel, Early conceptions of humor: varieties and issues, Chapter 1, pp. 3–39, In: J.H. Goldstein and P.E. McGhee, **The Psychology of Humor**, London: Academic Press, 1972.

14 C. Darwin, **Emotions in Man and Animals**, New York: Greenwood Press, Publishers, 1969.

15 R. Descartes, **Les Passions de L'âme** Paris, 1649, cited In: P. Keith-Spiegel, Early Conceptions of Humor: Varieties and Issues, Chapter 1, pp. 3–39, In: J.H. Goldstein and P.E. McGhee **The Psychology of Humor**, London: Academic Press, 1972.

16 T. Hobbes, **Leviathan** London: Crooke, 1651, cited In: P. Keith-Spiegel, Early Conceptions of Humor: Varieties and Issues, Chapter 1, pp. 3–39, In: J.H. Goldstein and P.E. McGhee, **The Psychology of Humor**, London: Academic Press, 1972.

17 Joubert (1579) cited in M. Eastman (1921) **The Sense of Humor**, New York: Scribner, cited In: P. Keith-Spiegel, Early Conceptions of Humor: Varieties and Issues, Chapter 1, pp. 3–39, In: J.H. Goldstein and P.E. McGhee, **The Psychology of Humor**, London: Academic Press, 1972.

18 C.P. Wilson, **Jokes: Form Content Use and Function**, London: Academic Press, 1979.

19 A.R. Radcliffe-Brown, **Structure and Function in Primitive Society**, New York: The Free Press, 1952, cited In: V.R. Robinson, **Humor and the Health Professions**, USA: Charles B. Slack, Inc, 1977.

20 D. Mitchell (ed), **A New Dictionary of Sociology**, 2nd edn, London: Routledge and Kegan Paul Ltd, 1981.

21 H. Kuper, Kinship among the Swazi, pp. 86–110. In: A.R. Radcliffe-Brown and D. Forde (eds) **African Systems of Kinship and Marriage**, London: Oxford University Press, 1975.

22 M. Fortes, Kinship and marriage among the Ashanti pp. 252–84. In: A.R. Radcliffe-Brown and D. Forde (eds), **African Systems of Kinship and Marriage**, London: Oxford University Press, 1975.

23 M. Gluckman, Kinship and marriage among the Lozi of Northern Rhodesia and the Zulu of Natal, pp. 166–206 In: A.R. Radcliffe-Brown and D. Forde, (eds), **African Systems of Kinship and Marriage**, London: Oxford University Press, 1975.

24 I. Shapera, Kinship and marriage among the Tswana, p. 140. In: A.R. Radcliffe-Brown and D. Forde (eds), **African Systems of Kinship and Marriage**, London: Oxford University Press, 1975.

25 A.J. Obrdlik, Gallows humor—a sociological phenomenon, **American Journal of Sociology**, 47: 709–16, 1942.

26 L. La Fave and R. Mannell, Does ethnic humor serve prejudice' **Journal of Communication**, 26: 120–3, 1976.

27 J. Revill, PMT sufferers ask comic Jim to join them, **Evening Standard**, 15 April, 1993.

28 N. Bruning, **Coping with Chemotherapy**, New York: The Dial Press, Doubleday and Company Inc, 1989.

29 N. Cousins, **Anatomy of an Illness as Perceived by the Patient**, New York: WW Norton and Company, 1979.

30 K. Fox Tennant, The effect of humor on the recovery rate of cataract patients: a pilot study, Chapter 13, pp. 245–51, In: L. Nahemow, K.A. McCluskey-Fawcett and P.E. McGhee (eds) **Humor and Aging**, London: Academic Press, 1986.

31 L.S. Kubie, The destructive potential of humor in psychotherapy, **The American Journal of Psychotherapy**, 127(7): 861–6, 1971.

32 R.B. Mancke, S. Maloney and M. West, Clowning: A healing process, **Health Education**, 5: 16–18, 1984.

33 J.F. Martin, Humor in therapy: an observational study. (University of Tennessee), **Dissertation Abstracts International**, 44(04): 1245-8, 1983.

34 C.W. Metcalf, Humor, life and death, **Oncology Nursing Forum**, 14(4): 19–21, 1987.

35 J. Napora, A study of the effects of a program of humorous activity on the subjective well-being of senior adults. (1984 University of Maryland Baltimore Professional Schools), **Dissertation Abstracts International**, 46(1): 276-A, 1985.

36 K.E. Peterson, The use of humor in AIDS prevention, in the treatment of HIV-positive persons, and in the remediation of caregiver burnout. Chapter 2 In: M.R. Seligson and K.E. Peterson (eds) **AIDS. Prevention and Treatment: Hope, Humor and Healing**, USA: Hemisphere Publishing Corporation, 1992.

37 R.E. Potter and N.J. Goodman, The implementation of laughter as a therapy facilitator with adult aphasics **Journal of Communication Disorders** 16: 41–8 1983.

38 N. Schmitt, Patients' perception of laughter in a rehabilitation hospital. **Rehabilitation Nursing,** 15(3): 143–6, 1990.

39 R.A. Martin and H.M. Lefcourt, Sense of humor as a moderator of the relation between stressors and moods, **Journal of Personality and Social Psychology,** 45(6): 1313–24, 1983.

40 R.H. Coombs and L.J. Goldman, Maintenance and discontinuity of coping mechanisms in an intensive care unit, **Social Problems,** 20: 342, 1973.

41 H. Mindness, The Use and Abuse of Humor in Psychotherapy, Chapter 15, pp. 331–41, In: A.J. Chapman and H.C. Foot, (eds), **Humor and Laughter: Theory, Research and Applications,** London: John Wiley and Sons, 1976.

42 R. Safranek and T. Schill, Coping with stress: does humor help? **Psychological Reports,** 51: 222, 1982.

43 M.E Bullock, The effects of humor on anxiety and divergent thinking in children (California School of Professional Psychology), **Dissertation Abstracts International,** 44(04): 1219-B, 1983.

44 N.F. Dixon, Humor: a cognitive alternative to stress? Chapter 18, pp 281–9, In: I.G. Sarason and C.D. Spielberger (eds) **Stress and Anxiety, Vol 10,** Washington: Hemisphere Publishing Corporation, 1980.

45 P. Nemeth, An investigation into the relationship between humor and anxiety. (United States International University), **Dissertation Abstracts International,** 40: 1378-B, 1979.

46 T.R. Shultz, Cognitive-developmental analysis of humour, Chapter 1, pp. 11–35, In: A.J. Chapman and H.C. Foot, **Humor and Laughter: Theory, Research and Applications,** London: John Wiley and Sons, 1976.

47 R.A. Martin and H.M. Lefcourt, Situational humor response questionnaire: quantitative measure of sense of humor **Journal of Personality and Social Psychology,** 47(1): 145–55 1984.

48 W.E. O'Connell, Freudian humour: the eupsychia of everyday life., Chapter 14, pp. 313–29, In: A.J. Chapman and H.C. Foot, **Humor and Laughter: Theory, Research and Applications,** London: John Wiley and Sons, 1976.

49 J.M. Simon, Humor and the older adult: implications for nursing. **Journal of Advanced Nursing,** 13: 441–6, 1988.

50 W.F. Fry, Psychodynamics of sexual humor: sex and the elderly, **Medical Aspects of Human Sexuality,** 10: 140–48, 1976.

51 D.R. Mettee, E.S. Hrelec and P.C. Wilkens, Humor as an interpersonal asset and liability, **The Journal of Social Psychology,** 85: 51–64, 1971.

52 G.A. Fine, Sociological approaches to the study of humor, Chapter 8, pp. 159–81, In: P.E. McGhee and J.H. Goldstein (eds), **Handbook of Humor Research, Volume 1, Basic Issues,** New York: Springer-Verlag, 1983.

53 J.M. Davis and A. Farina, Humor appreciation as social communication, **Journal of Personality and Social Psychology,** 15(2): 175–8, 1970.

54 W.H. Martineau, A model of the social functions of humor, Chapter 5, pp. 101–25, In: J.H. Goldstein and P.E. McGhee, **The Psychology of Humor**, London: Academic Press, 1972.

55 A. Dundes, At ease, disease—AIDS jokes as sick humor, **American Behavioral Scientist**, 30(1): 72–81, 1987.

56 G. Jefferson, H. Sacks and E. Schegloff, Notes on laughter in the pursuit of intimacy, Chapter 7, pp. 152–216, In: G. Button and J.R.E. Lee, **Talk and Social Organisation**, Clevedon, Philadelphia: Multilingual Matters Ltd, 1987.

57 R.L. Coser, Some social functions of laughter. A study of humor in a hospital setting, **Human Relations**, XII(2): 171–82, 1959.

58 G. Jefferson, A technique for inviting laughter and its subsequent acceptance declination, pp. 79–95, In: G. Psathas, **Everyday Language. Studies in Ethnomethodology**, New York: Irvington Publications Inc, 1979.

59 J. Porteous, Humor as a process of defense: the evolution of laughing. **Humor–International Journal of Humor Research**, 1(1): 63–80, 1988.

60 M. Godkewitsch, Physiological and verbal indices of arousal in rated humour, Chapter 6, pp. 117–38, In: A.J. Chapman and H.C. Foot, **Humor and Laughter: Theory, Research and Applications**, London: John Wiley and Sons, 1976.

61 R. Langevin and H.I. Day, Physiological correlates of Humor, Chapter 6, pp. 129–41, In: J.H. Goldstein and P.E. McGhee, **The Psychology of Humor**, London: Academic Press, 1972.

62 W.F. Fry and W.M. Savin, Mirthful laughter and blood pressure, **Humor-International Journal of Humor Research**, 1(1): 49–62, 1988.

63 D.E. Berylne, Humor and its kin, Chapter 2, pp. 43–60, In: J.H. Goldstein and P.E. McGhee, **The Psychology of Humor**, London: Academic Press, 1972.

64 K.M. Dillon, B. Minchoff and K.H. Baker, Positive emotional states and enhancement of the immune system, **International Journal of Psychiatry in Medicine**, 15(1): 13–18 1985.

65 L.S. Berk, S.A. Tan, S.L. Nehlsen-Cannarella, B.J. Napier, J.W. Lee, J.E. Lewis, R.W. Hubbard, W.C. Eby and W.F. Fry, Mirth modulates adrenocorticomedullary activity: suppression of cortisol and epinephrine, **Clinical Research**, 36(1): 121A, 1988.

66 L.S. Berk, S.A. Tan, S.L. Nehlsen-Cannarella, B.J. Napier, J.E. Lewis, J.W. Lee, W.C. Eby and W.F. Fry, Humor associated laughter decreases cortisol and increases spontaneous lymphocyte blastogenesis, **Clinical Research**, 36(3): 435A, 1988.

67 R. Cogan, D. Cogan, W. Waltz and M. McCue, Effects of laughter and relaxation on discomfort thresholds, **Journal of Behavioral Medicine**, 10(2): 139–44, 1987.

68 J.P. Emerson, Negotiating the serious import of humor, **Sociometry**, 32: 169–81, 1969.

69 A.L. Crane, Why sickness can be a laughing matter, **Registered Nurse**, 50: 41–2, 1987.

70 V.R. Robinson, Humor in Nursing, Chapter 7, pp. 129–51, In: C.E. Carlson and B. Blackwell (eds), 2nd edn, **Behavioral Concepts and Nursing Intervention**, USA: JB Lippincott Company, 1970.

71 D. Spiegel, P. Keith-Spiegel, J. Abrahams, and L. Kranitz, Humor and suicide: Favorite jokes of suicidal patients, **Journal of Consulting and Clinical Psychology**, 33(4): 504–5, 1969.

72 S. Van Zandt and C. LaFont, Can a laugh a day keep the doctor away? **Journal of Practical Nursing**, 9: 33–35, 1985.

73 G. Ferraro Donnelly, Under stress? Try laughing it off, **Registered Nurse**, 4: 41–3, 1981.

74 D. Burton Leiber, Laughter and humor in critical care. **Dimensions of Critical Care Nursing**, 5(3): 162–70, 1986.

75 L. Gibson, Comic relief, **Nursing Times**, 86(38): 50–1, 1990.

76 R.L. Reynes and M.D. Allen, Humor in psychotherapy: A view, **American Journal of Psychotherapy**, XLI(2): 260–70, 1987.

77 S. Sands, The use of humor in psychotherapy, **Psychoanalytic Review**, 71(3): 441–60, 1984.

78 J.E. Heuscher, The role of humor and folklore themes in psychotherapy, **American Journal of Psychiatry**, 137(12): 1546–1549, 1980.

Further Reading

K.M. Avant, Humor and self-disclosure. **Psychological Reports**, 50: 253–4, 1982.
This study examines the relationships between humour and self disclosure of 28 male and 59 female undergraduates. Humour was measured by a 5-choice continuum and self-disclosure by a questionnaire. Significant relationships were found between perceived humour and self-disclosure. This is a short paper of interest to those who prefer a more positivist or 'quantitative' approach.

R.A. Baron, Aggression-inhibiting influence of sexual humor. **Journal of Personality and Social Psychology**, 2: 189–97, 1978.
Forty-eight undergraduate males were studied using a quasi-experimental design to test the hypothesis that prior exposure to sexual humour would reduce the level of aggression directed by angry individuals against the person who had previously provoked them. Results indicated that exposure to exploitative sexual humour, but not exposure to non-exploitative sexual humour, significantly reduced the strength of subjects' later attacks against the victim.

D.W. Black, Laughter. **Journal of the American Medical Association**, 252(21): 2295–3014, 1984.
A brief review which includes an anatomical, neurological, psychological and developmental approach to laughter.

A.J Chapman and H.C. Foot, **Humor and Laughter: Theory, Research and Applications**, London: John Wiley and Sons, 1976.
This is a research based text which is good for details but not always easy for a non-researcher to read. The book contains psychotherapy, sociological, psychological and physiological approaches.

N. Cousins, **Head First. The Biology of Hope,** New York: E.P. Dutton, 1989.
An interesting and easy read, providing insight into Cousins' beliefs and experiences. The text also includes some useful clinical references.

W.F Fry and W.A. Salameh, (eds) **Handbook of Humor and Psychotherapy. Advances in the Clinical Use of Humor,** Sarasota, Florida: Professional Resources Exchange, Inc, 1987.
Some interesting research and ancedotal evidence of the use of laughter and humour. The text includes a clinical bibliography, although many of the references are pre-1980s.

J.H. Goldstein and P.E. McGhee, **The Psychology of Humor,** London: Academic Press, 1972.
Another research-based text that may be of more interest to researchers. Includes sociological, physiological and psychological perspectives.

A.H. Hunt, Humor as a nursing intervention, **Cancer Nursing,** 16 (1): 34–9, 1993.
This provides a useful overview and discusses the results of six research studies in which health care professionals used humour as a treatment protocol. Includes 25 references.

J. Mallett, Use of humour and laughter in patient care, **British Journal of Nursing,** 2(3): 172–4, 1993.
This paper briefly introduces some concepts from preliminary analysis of data from audiovisual tapes of humour used between nurses and patients in clinical settings.

P.E. McGhee and J.H. Goldstein, (eds) **Handbook of Humor Research Volume 1 Basic Issues,** New York: Springer-Verlag, 1983.
A research based book which incorporates anthropological, physiological and sociological perspectives on humour.

L. Nahemow, Humor as a data base for the study of aging, Ch. 1 pp. 3–26 In: L. Nahemow, K.A. McCluskey-Fawcett and P.E. McGhee, **Humor and Aging,** London: Academic Press, 1986.
Contains many references but readers need to be interested in theory to read this.

O. Nevo and J. Shapiro, Use of humor in managing clinical anxiety, **Journal of Dentistry for Children,** 53(2): 97–100, 1986.
This paper provides the results of interviews with 10 specialists in paediatric dentistry regarding their use of humour. This would be of interest to a clinician but may not be detailed enough for the researcher wanting to replicate the study.

H.R. Pollio, R. Mers and W. Lucchesi, Humor, laughter, and smiling: some preliminary observations of funny behaviours, Ch. 11, pp. 211–39, In: J.H. Goldstein and P.E. McGhee, **The Psychology of Humor,** London: Academic Press, 1972.
The aim of this research was to describe laughter quantitatively (including amplitude and duration of bursts of laughter) using an oscillographic record. Data of audience laughter was collected by recording at an amateur theatre production and a local film on different nights, and a television comedy programme (canned laughter). The analysis considers the differences between the groups.

F.J. Prerost, Evaluating the systematic use of humor in psychotherapy with adolescents, **Journal of Adolescents,** 7(3): 267–76, 1984.
This paper describes the use of Humourous Imagery Situation Technique (HIST) in psychotherapy on adolscents. A case history is discussed.

S.L. Ragan, Verbal play and multiple goals in the gynaecological exam interaction, **Journal of Language and Social Psychology**, 9(1–2): 67–84, 1990.

A good paper which discusses the use of humour between nurse practitioners and patients during gynaecological examinations. Interesting for both clinicians and researchers.

E.M. Scott, Humor and the alcoholic patient: a beginning study, **Alcoholism Treatment Quarterly**, 6(2): 29–30, 1989.

A questionnaire was used to collect data on humour from 120 individuals applying for help at an alcoholic outpatient agency. The results indicate an 'overwhelming endorsement' that humour be an aspect of psychotherapy. An interesting study that is easily understandable.

Appendix:
Useful addresses and telephone numbers

Every effort has been made to ensure that the following addresses and telephone numbers are current and correct, but the Publishers will be most grateful for information regarding any recent changes, along with suggestions for new inclusions in future editions. Please also note that the addresses included below do not necessarily imply their recommendation by either the Editors or the Publishers: individuals are therefore directed to consult the relevant validating bodies, and to the advice given in Section 5 of the Appendix.

Contents

Section I:
Professional Organisations and Associations

Association of General Practitioners of Natural Medicine
30 Nigel House
Portpool Lane
London EC1N 7UR
Tel: 071 405 2781

Association for Holistic Medicine
Sundrum Castle
Sundrum by Ayr
Scotland KA6 5JY
Tel: 0292 570889

Association of Holistic Therapies
39 Prestbury Road
Attville
Cheltenham
Gloucestershire GL2 2PT
Tel: 0242 512601

Association of Natural Medicines
27 Braintree Road
Witham
Essex CM8 2DD
Tel: 0376 511069

British Complementary Medicine Association
St Charles Hospital
Exmoor Street
London W10 6DZ
Tel: 081 964 1205

British Complementary Medical Examination Board
PO Box 194
London SE16 1QZ
Tel: 071 237 5165

British Council of Complementary Medicine
PO Box 194
London SE16 1QZ
Tel: 071 237 5165

British Holistic Health Services Association
100 Wigmore Street
London W1H 0AE
Tel: 071 486 0431

British Holistic Medical Association
St Marylebone Parish Church
Marylebone Road
London NW1 5LT
Tel: 071 262 5299

British Medical Association
BMA House
Tavistock Square
London WC1H 9JP
Tel: 071 387 4499

British Register of Complementary Practitioners
PO Box 194
London SE16 1QZ
Tel: 071 237 5165

City and Guilds of London Institute
76 Portland Place
London W1N 4AA

Confederation of Beauty Therapy and Cosmetology
Suite 5
Wolseley House
Oriel Road
Cheltenham
Gloucestershire

Council for Complementary and Alternative Medicine
Suite 1
19a Cavendish Square
London W1M 9AD
Tel: 071 409 1440

Council for Professions Supplementary to Medicine
Park House
184 Kennington Park Road
London SE11 4BU
Tel: 071 582 0866

Health Practitioners' Association (Incorp. Guild of Practitioners of Natural Therapies)
187a Worlds End
Chelsfield
Kent BR6 6AU
Tel: 0689 31211

Institute for Complementary Medicine
PO Box 194
London SE16 1QZ
Tel: 071 237 5165

Institute of Holistic Therapies
486 Fulham Road
London SW6 5NH
Tel: 081 540 1743

ITEC-International Therapy Examination Council
16 Avenue Place
Harrogate
North Yorkshire HG2 7PJ

International Guild of Natural Medicine Practitioners & Register
3 Chatsworth Road
Luton
Bedfordshire LU4 8AS
Tel: 0582 585390

Marylebone Centre Trust
Regent's College
Regent's Park
London NW1 4NS
Tel: 071 487 7415

National Consultative Council for Alternative and Complementary Medicine
39 Prestbury Road
Cheltenham
Gloucestershire GL52 2PT

National Foundation for Holistic Medicine
Suncourt Leafdale
The Lough
Cork
Ireland
Tel: 010 353 219 64470

Royal Society of Medicine
1 Wimpole Street
London W1M 8AE
Tel: 071 408 2119
Telex: 298902 ROYMED G

Society of Biological Medicine
398 Uxbridge Road
Hatch End
Pinner
Middlesex HA5 4HP
Tel: 081 428 4333

Society of Holistic Practitioners
Sundrum Castle
Sundrum by Ayr
Scotland KA4 5JY
Tel: 0292 570889

Society of Registered Holistic Medicine Practitioners
54 Cardington Square
Hounslow West
Middlesex TW4 6AJ
Tel: 081 570 3693

Society of Students of Holistic Health
160 Upper Fant Road
Maidstone
Kent ME16 8DJ
Tel: 0662 29231

Section 2:
Research bodies

Specific research bodies, for individual therapies, are listed in Section 4 of the Appendix.

Centre for Complementary Health Studies
University of Exeter
Streatham Court
Rennes Drive
Exeter EX4 4PU
Tel: 0392 433828/263263

Centre for Dream Research
8 Willow Road
London NW3
Tel: 071 794 8717

Centre for Medical Research
Mantell Building
University of Sussex
Falmer
Brighton BN1 9RF
Tel: 0273 606755 ext 3654

Confederation of Healing Organizations
The Red and White House
113 High Street
Berkhampstead
Hertfordshire HP4 2DJ
Tel: 0442 870660

Health Research Unit
Department of Psychology
Surrey University
Guildford
Surrey GU2 5XH
Tel: 0483 571281

Henry Doubleday Research Association
Ryton Gardens
Ryton-on-Dunsmore
Coventry CV8 3LG
Tel: 0203 303517

Holistic Health Research Network
18 March St
Strathbungo
Glasgow G41 2PX
Tel: 041 424 0603

Institute for Complementary Medicine
PO Box 194
London SE16 1QZ
Tel: 071 237 5165

Koestler Foundation
484 Kings Road
London SW10
Tel: 071 376 5959

Medical Research Council
20 Park Crescent
London W1N 4AL
Tel: 071 636 5422

Natural Therapeutic Research Trust
Gislingham
Near Eye
Suffolk IP23 8JG
Tel: 037983 527

Research Council for Complementary Medicine (RCCM)
5th Floor
60 Great Ormond Street
London WC1 3JF
Tel: 071 833 8897

Society for Psychical Research
1 Adam and Eve Mews
London W8 6UG
Tel: 071 937 8984

Section 3:
Schools and colleges

Academy of Health
80 Portland Road
Bournemouth
Dorset BH9 1NQ
Tel: 0202 529793

Arnauld-Taylor Education Ltd
James House
Okelbrook Mill
Newent
Gloucestershire GL18 1HD
Tel: 0531 821875

Brighton Natural Health Centre
27 Regent Street
Brighton BN1 1UL
Tel: 0273 600010

Centre for the Study of Complementary Medicine
51 Bedford Place
Southampton
Hampshire SO1 2DG
Tel: 0703 334752

College of Alternative Medicine and Science
Little Acre
Marine Drive
Widemouth Bay
Bude
Cornwall EX23 0AQ
Tel: 028885 428

College of Healing
Runnings Park
Croft Bank
West Malvern
Worcestershire WR14 4DU
Tel: 0684 565253

College of Holistic Medicine
Old Hall
East Bergholt
Colchester CO7 6TG

College of Natural Medicine
38 Nigel House
Portpool Lane
London EC1
Tel: 071 405 2781

College of Natural Therapy
133 Gatley Road
Gatley
Cheadle
Cheshire SK8 4PD

Edinburgh School of Natural Therapy
2 London Street
Edinburgh EH3 6NA
Tel: 031 557 3901

Findhorn Foundation
Cluny Hill College
Forres
Scotland IV36 0RD
Tel: 0309 72288

Ffynnonwen Natural Therapy Centre
Llangwyryfon
Aberystwyth
Dyfed SY23 4EY
Tel: 09747 376

Gablecroft College of Natural Therapy
Church Street
Whittington
Oswestry
Shropshire S11 4DT
Tel: 0691 658631

Health and Beauty Therapy Training Board
PO Box 21
Bognor Regis
West Sussex PO22 7PS
Tel: 0243 860339

Holistic Healing Centre
92 Sheering Road
Old Harlow
Essex CM17 0JW

Hoths School for Holistic Therapy
39 Prestbury Road
Pittville
Cheltenham
Gloucestershire GL2 2PT
Tel: 0242 512601

and

1 Hall Lane
Aylestone
Leicestershire LE2 8SF
Tel: 0533 837305

Information and Study Centre for Alternative Medicine
64 Bower Mount Road
Maidstone
Kent ME16 8AT
Tel: 0622 54858

Institute of Bioenergetic Medicine
103 North Road
Poole
Dorset BH14 0LT
Tel: 0202 733762

London Sufi Centre
21 Lancaster Road
London W11 1QL
Tel: 071 221 1064/3215

Maperton Trust
Wincanton
Somerset BA9 8EH
Tel: 0963 32651

Moorlands Natural Medicine Teaching Centre
Moorlands
24 South Road
Newton Abbot
Devon TQ12 1HQ
Tel: 0626 65493

Natural Healing Centre
27 Braintree Road
Witham
Essex CM8 2BS
Tel: 0376 511069

Natural Health Centre Training School
33 Bromley Road
Lytham St Annes
Lancashire FY8 1PQ

Natural Therapeutic Centre
Gislingham
Near Eye
Suffolk
Tel: 0379 83527

Polytechnic of Central London
115 New Cavendish Street
London W1M 8JS
Tel: 071 580 2020

Raworth College for Sports Therapy and Natural Medicines
Smallburgh
Beare Green
Dorking
Surrey RH5 4QA
Tel: 0306 712623

Richardson Clinic
Westgate
Heckmondwicke
West Yorkshire
Tel: 0924 402763

School of Complementary Medicine
9 Sharpleshall Street
London NW1 8YN
Tel: 071 586 1263

Section 4:
Addresses for specific therapies

The addresses in this section cover organizations, research bodies, and a selection of training institutions and are listed in alphabetical order by therapy.

ACUPRESSURE AND SHIATSU

British School of Oriental Therapy & Movement
46 Whitton Road
Twickenham
Middx TW1 1BS
Tel: 081 744 1974

British School of Shiatsu
East West Centre
188 Old Street
London EC1V 9BP
Tel: 071 251 0831

British Shiatsu Council
121 Sheen Road
Richmond
Surrey TW9 1YJ
Tel: 081 852 1080

European Shiatsu School
Central Administration
High Banks
Lockeridge
Near Malborough
Wiltshire SN8 4EQ
Tel: 0672 86363

Glasgow School of Shiatsu
Contact: Elaine Liecht: MA MRSS
19 Langside Park
Kilbarchan
Renfrewshire PA10 2EP
Tel: 05057 4657
(Courses are taught at the Complementary Medicine Centre
17 Queens Crescent
Glasgow G4)

Healing/Shiatsu Education Centre
The Orchard
Lower Maescoed
Pontrilas
Herefordshire HR2 0HP
Tel: 087387 207

London Centre for Yoga and Shiatsu Studies
Department Tac
49B Onslow Gardens
London N10 3JY
Tel: 081 444 0103

London College of Massage & Shiatsu
21 Portland Place
London W1N 3AF
Tel: 071 636 9543

The London College of Shiatsu
LCS
1 Central Park Lodge
54-58 Bolsover Street
London W1P 7HL
Tel: 071 383 2619

Nine Needles College of Oriental Medicine
121 Sheen Road
Richmond
Surrey TW9 1YJ
Tel: 081 940 8892

Shen Tao Foundation
Middle Piccadilly Natural Healing Centre
Holwell
Sherborne
Dorset
Tel: 09632 3468

The Shiatsu Society
5 Foxcote
Wokingham
Berkshire RG11 3PG

ACUPUNCTURE

Acupuncture & Chinese Herbal Practitioners' Training College
1037b Finchley Road
Golders Green
London NW11 7ES
Tel: 081 455 5508

Acupuncture Foundation & Teaching Clinic
1st Floor
151-153 Clapham High Street
London SW4
Tel: 071 267 1380

Acupuncture Research Association
118 Foley Road
Claygate
Esher
Surrey KT10 0NA
Tel: 0372 64171

Association of Irish Acupuncturists
81 Merrion Road
Ballsbridge
Dublin
Eire
Tel: 0001 692934

Association of Western Acupuncture
Burton Manor College
Burton
Wirral
Cheshire L64 5SJ
Tel: 051 336 5172

British Acupuncture Association and Register
34 Alderney Street
London SW1V 4EU
Tel: 071 834 1012

British Academy of Western Acupuncture
Burton Manor College
Burton
Wirral
Cheshire L64 5SJ
Tel: 051 336 5172

British College of Acupuncture
8 Hunter Street
London WC1N 1BN
Tel: 071 833 8164

British Medical Acupuncture Society
69 Chancery Lane
London WC1

Chung San Acupuncture School
15 Porchester Gardens
London W2 4DB
Tel: 071 727 6778

Chung San Acupuncture Society
15 Porchester Gardens
London W2 4DB
Tel: 071 727 6778/228 1036

College of Holistic Therapies
Administration Secretary
Suncourt Leafdale
The Lough
Cork
Ireland
Tel: 021 964470

College of Traditional Chinese Acupuncture
Tao House
Queensway
Leamington Spa
Warwickshire CV31 3LZ
Tel: 0926 422121

Council for Acupuncture
Panther House
38 Mount Pleasant
London WC1X 0AP
Tel: 071 837 8026

Electroacupuncture according to Voll Society of Britain and Ireland
400 Uxbridge Road
Hatch End
Pinner
Middlesex HA5 4HP
Tel: 081 428 4435

Fook Sang Acupuncture and Chinese Herbal Practitioners' Training College UK
1037b Finchley Road
Golders Green
London
NW11 7ES
Tel: 081 455 5508

International College of Oriental Medicine
Green Hedges House
Green Hedges Avenue
East Grinstead
West Sussex RH19 1DZ

The Liu Academy of Traditional Chinese Medicine
13 Gunnersbury Avenue
Ealing Common
London W5 3XD
Tel: 081 993 2549/992 2611

London School of Acupuncture and Traditional Chinese Medicine
36 Featherstone Street
London EC1Y 8QX
Tel: 071 490 0513

Nine Needles College of Oriental Medicine
121 Sheen Road
Richmond
Surrey TW9 1YJ
Tel: 081 940 8892

Northern College of Acupuncture
124 Acomb Road
York YO2 4EY
Tel: 0904 785120

ALEXANDER TECHNIQUE

Alexander Technique Training Centre
Fox Hole
Dartington
Devon TQ9 6EJ
Tel: 0803 864218

Constructive Teaching Centre
18 Landsdowne Road
London W11 3LL
Tel: 071 727 7222

North London Alexander School
10 Elmfoot Avenue
London NW11 0RR
Tel: 081 455 3938

Professional Association of Alexander Teachers
14 Kingsland
Jesmond
Newcastle Upon Tyne
Tyne and Wear NE2 3AL
Tel: 091 281 8032

Society of Teachers of Alexander Technique
10 London House
266 Fulham Road
London SW10 9EL
Tel: 071 351 0828

The Alexander Technique Teaching Centre
188 Old Street
London EC1V 9BP
Tel: 071 250 3038

ALLERGY THERAPY AND CLINICAL ECOLOGY

Action Against Allergy
43 The Downs
London SW10 8HG
Tel: 081 947 5082

British Society of Allergy and Environmental Medicine
Burghwood Clinic
34 Brighton Road
Banstead
Surrey SM17 1BS
Tel: 0737 361177/352245

Institute of Allergy Therapists
Fynnonwen
Llangwyryfon
Aberystwyth
Dyfed SY23 4EY
Tel: 09747 376

AROMATHERAPY

Armould-Taylor Education Ltd
James House
Oakelbrook Hill
Newent
Gloucestershire GL18 1HD

Aromatherapy and Beauty Therapy Training Centre
2 Church Close
Andover
Hampshire
Tel: 0264 52935

Aromatherapy Associates
7 Wardo Avenue
Fulham
London SW6
Tel: 071 371 0465

Aromatherapy Organizations Council
3 Laymers Close
Bray Carook
Market Harborough LE16 8LL
Tel: 0455 615466

**Aromatherapy School Promotion
Centre**
The Natural Clinic
Bretland House
1 Bretland Road
Rusthall
Tunbridge Wells
Kent TN4 8PB

Aromatherapy World
c/o ISPA
41 Leicester Road
Leicestershire LE10 1LW

**Association of Tisserand
Aromatherapists**
PO Box 746
Brighton
East Sussex BN1 3BN
Tel: 0273 206640

**Bournemouth School of Massage and
Aromatherapy**
14 Greenwood
Bournemouth BH9 2LH
Tel: 0202 513838

Institute of Clinical Aromatherapy
22 Bromley Road
Catford
London SE6 2TP
Tel: 081 690 2149

**International Federation of
Aromatherapists**
Dept. of Continuing Education
The Royal Masonic Hospital
Ravenscourt Park
London W6 0TN
Tel: 081 846 8066

**International Journal of
Aromatherapy**
65 Church Road
Hove
East Sussex BN3 2BD

**The International Society of
Professional Aromatherapists**
41 Leicester Road
Hinckley
Leicestershire LE10 1LW
Tel: 0455 637987

London School of Aromatherapy
PO Box 780
London NW5 1DY
Tel: 071 328 9504

**London School of Herbology &
Aromatherapy**
54A Gloucester Road
London NW1 8JD

**Micheline Arcier Aromatherapy
School**
7 William Street
Knightsbridge
London SW1X 9HL
Tel: 071 235 6545

Purple Flame School of Aromatherapy
61 Clinton Lane
Kenilworth
Warwickshire CV8 1AS

Register of Qualified Aromatherapists
54a Gloucester Avenue
London NW1 8JD

Shirley Price Aromatherapy Ltd
Wesley House
Stockwell Head
Hinckley
Leicestershire LE10 1RD
Tel: 0455 615466/615436

Tisserand Aromatherapy Institute
65 Church Road
Hove
Sussex
Tel: 0273 206640

ART THERAPY AND THE ARTS

The Arts Council
105 Piccadilly
London W1V 0AU

The British Association of Art Therapists Ltd
11a Richmond Road
Brighton
Sussex BN2 3RL

The Centre on Environments for Handicap
126 Albert Street
London NW1 7NF

Council for Music in Hospital
340 Lower Road
Little Bookham
Surrey KT23 4EF

Live Music Now
38 Wigmore Street
London W1H 9DF

Royal Ballet/Royal Opera House Education Department
Royal Opera House
Covent Garden
London WC2E 7QA

CHIROPRACTIC

Anglo-European College of Chiropractic
13-15 Parkwood Road
Boscombe
Bournemouth
Dorset BH5 2DF
Tel: 0202 431 021

British Chiropractic Association
Premier House
Greycoat Place
London SW1P 1SB
Tel: 071 222 8866

European Chiropractic Union
Ahlgade 3
4300 Holbeak
Denmark
Tel: 010 45 3 431192

Institute of Pure Chiropractic
PO Box 126
Oxford OX2 8RH
Tel: 0865 246687

McTimoney School of Chiropractic
PO Box 127
Oxford OX1 1HH
Tel: 0865 246786

Scottish Chiropractic Association
12 Walker Street
Edinburgh 3
Scotland
Tel: 031 225 7743

Witney School of Chiropractic
PO Box 69
Witney
Oxfordshire OX8 5YD

CHINESE AND ORIENTAL MEDICINE

International Register of Oriental Medicine
Green Hedges House
Green Hedges Avenue
East Grinstead
West Sussex RH19 1DZ
Tel: 0342 313106/7

Irish College of Traditional Chinese Medicine
100 Marlborough Road
Donnybrook
Dublin 4
Republic of Ireland
Tel: 0865 772560

Liu Clinics of Traditional Medicine
13 Gunnersbury Avenue
Ealing Common
London W5
Tel: 081 993 2549/992 2611

Professional Register of Traditional Chinese Medicine
17 Leinster Road West
Rathmines
Dublin 6
Republic of Ireland
Tel: 0001 978906

Register of Traditional Chinese Medicine
19 Trinity Road
London N2 8JJ
Tel: 081 883 8431

School of T'ai-chi Ch'uan Centre for Healing
5 Tavistock Place
London WC1
Tel: 081 886 9664

Traditional Acupuncture Society
1 The Ridgeway
Stratford-Upon-Avon
Warwickshire CV37 9JL
Tel: 0789 298798

COLOUR/LIGHT THERAPY

Aura Soma
Dev Aura
Little London
Tetford
Lincolnshire LN9 6QL
Tel: 065883 781

Hygeia College of Colour Therapy
Brook House
Avening
Tetbury
Gloucestershire GL8 8NS
Tel: 045383 2150

Hygeia Studios Colour-Light Art Research Ltd
Brook House
Avening
Tetbury
Gloucestershire GL8 8NS
Tel: 045383 2150

International Association of Colour Healers
21 Portland Place
London W1N 3AF
Tel: 071 636 9543

International Association of Colour Therapists
Brook House
Avening
Tetbury
Gloucestershire GL8 8NS
Tel: 045383 2150

Universal Colour Healers
67 Farm Crescent
Wexham Court
Slough
Berkshire SL2 5TQ
Tel: 0753 76913

Universal Colour Healers Research Foundation
67 Farm Crescent
Wexham Court
Slough
Berkshire SL2 5TQ
Tel: 0753 76913

CRANIO-SACRAL THERAPY

College of Cranio-Sacral Therapy (CCST)
160 Upper Fant Road
Maidstone
Kent ME16 8DJ
Tel: 0622 729231

Cranial Osteopathic Association
478 Baker Street
Enfield
Middlesex EN1 3QS
Tel: 081 367 5561

Craniosacral Therapy Educational Trust
29 Dollis Park
Finchley
London N3 1HJ
Tel: 081 349 0297

CRYSTAL/ELECTRO-CRYSTAL THERAPY

Academy of Crystal and Natural Awareness
Crystal House
4 Bridgwater Road
Bleadon
Weston-Super-Mare BS24 0BG
Tel: 0934 815083

Association of Crystal Healing Therapists
5 Sunneymede Vale
Holcombe Brook
Bury
Lancashire BL0 944
Tel: 020488 3482

Crystal Research Foundation
37 Bromley Road
St Annes-on-Sea
Lancashire FY8 1PQ
Tel: 0253 723735

Electrocrystal Therapy Research and Development
117 Long Drive South
Ruislip
Middlesex HA4 0HL
Tel: 081 841 1716

Institute of Crystal and Gem Therapists
Anubis House
Bullens Courtyard
Mill Lane Mews
Ashby de la Zouch
Leicestershire LE6 5HP
Tel: 0530 510864

School of Electro-Crystal Therapy
117 Long Drive
South Ruislip
Middlesex HA4 0HL
Tel: 081 841 1716

Wholistic Research Company
Bright Haven
Robins Lane
Lolworth
Cambridge CB3 8HH
Tel: 0954 781074

DANCE/DRAMA THERAPY

The Actors' Institute
137 Goswell Road
London EC1
Tel: 071 251 8178

DIETARY/NUTRITION THERAPY

Biosocial Therapy Association
126 High Road
East Finchley
London N2
Tel: 081 444 8694

The British Dietetic Association
7th Floor
Elizabeth House
22 Suffolk Street
Queensway
Birmingham B1 1LS

British Nutrition Foundation
15 Belgrave Square
London SW1X 8PG
Tel: 071 235 4904

British Society for Nutritional Medicine
PO Box 3AP
London W1A 3AP
Tel: 071 436 8532

College of Nutritional Medicine
East Bank
New Church Road
Smithills
Greater Manchester BL1 5QP
Tel: 0204 492 550

Dietary Therapy Society
33 Priory Gardens
London N6 5QU
Tel: 081 341 7260

Foundation for Applied Nutrition
133 Gately Road
Gatley
Cheadle
Cheshire SK8 4PD
Tel: 061 428 4980

Health Education Authority
78 New Oxford St
London
WC1A 1AH

Institute for Optimum Nutrition
5 Jerdan Place
Fulham
London SW6 1BE
Tel: 071 385 7984/8673

Jewish Vegetarian Society
Bet Teva
855 Finchley Road
London NW11 8DX
Tel: 081 455 0692

McCarrison Society
24 Paddington Street
London W1M 4DR
Tel: 071 935 3924

Natural Flow
Burwash Common
East Sussex TN19 7LX
Tel: 0435 882482

Nutrition Society
Grosvenor Gardens House
35-37 Grosvenor Gardens
London SW1W 0BS
Tel: 071 821 1243

Vegan Society
33-35 George Street
Oxford OX1 2AY
Tel: 0865 722166

Vegetarian Society
Parkdale
Dunham Road
Altrincham
Cheshire WA14 4QG
Tel: 061 928 0793

HEALING

Association for Therapeutic Healers
c/o Elizabeth St John
Flat 5
54-56 Neal Street
Covent Garden
London WC2
Tel: 071 240 0176

Atlanteans
Runnings Park
Croft Bank
West Malvern
Worcestershire WR14 4BP
Tel: 0684 565253

**British Alliance of Healing
Associations**
26 Highfield Avenue
Herne Bay
Kent CT6 6LM
Tel: 0227 373804

**Churches Council for Health and
Healing**
17 Marylebone Road
London NW1 5LT
Tel: 071 486 9644

College of Healing
Runnings Park
Croft Bank
West Malvern
Worcestershire WR14 4BP
Tel: 0684 565253

College of Psychic Studies
The College
16 Queensbury Place
London SW7 2EB
Tel: 071 589 3292/3

College of Psychotherapeutics
White Lodge
Stockland Green Road
Speldhurst
Tunbridge Wells
Kent TN3 0TT

**Confederation of Healing
Organizations**
The Red and White House
113 High Street
Berkhamstead
Hertfordshire HP4 2DJ
Tel: 0442 870660

Fellowship of Erasmus
The Bungalow
Tollemache Farm
Main Road
Offton
Ipswich
Suffolk IP8 4RT
Tel: 047333 217

**Greater World Christian Spiritual
Association**
3 Conway Street
Fitzrovia
London W1P 5HA
Tel: 071 436 7555

Guild of Spiritual Healers
36 Newmarket
Otley
West Yorkshire LS21 3AE
Tel: 0943 462708

Guild of St Raphael
St Marylebone Parish Church
Marylebone Road
London NW1 5LT
Tel: 071 935 6374 ext 127

**Harry Edwards Spiritual Healing
Sanctuary**
Burrows Lea
Shere
Guildford
Surrey GU5 9QG
Tel: 048641 2054

Health and Healing Committee
United Reform Church
84 Tavistock Place
London WC1H 9RT
Tel: 071 837 7661

**Institute for Advanced Health
Research**
51 The Park
Yeovil
Somerset BA20 1DF
Tel: 0935 29015

**Jewish Association of Spiritual
Healers**
10 Wollaton Road
Ferndown
Dorset BH22 8Q

Maitreya School of Healing
37 Third Avenue
Bexhill-on-Sea
East Sussex TN40 2PA
Tel: 0424 211450

**National Federation of Spiritual
Healers**
Old Manor Farm Studio
Church St
Sunbury-on-Thames
Middlesex TW16 6RG
Tel: 09327 83164/5

Prometheus School of Healing
152 Penistone Road
Huddersfield
West Yorkshire
Tel: 0484 602993

Spiritual Venturers Association
72 Pasture Road
Goole
North Humberside
Tel: 0405 69119

Spiritual Association of Great Britain
33 Belgrave Square
London SW1X 8QL
Tel: 071 235 3351

Spiritualists' National Union
Redwoods
Standsted Hall
Standsted Mountfitchet
Essex CM24 8UD
Tel: 0279 816363

Sufi Healing Order of Great Britain
10 Beauchamp Avenue
Leamington Spa
Warwickshire CU32 5TA
Tel: 0926 422388

Westbank Healing & Teaching Centre
Strathmiglo
Fife
Scotland KY14 7QP

White Eagle Lodge
New Lands
Brewells Lane
Rake
Liss
Hampshire GU33 7HY
Tel: 0730 893300

World Federation of Healing
6 Whitworth House
Buckhurst Road
Bexhill-on-Sea
East Sussex TN40 1UA
Tel: 0424 214457

HERBAL MEDICINE (PHYTOTHERAPY)

Anglo-European School of Herbalism
40 Stokewood Road
Bournemouth BH3 7NE
Tel: 0202 529793

College of Herbs and Natural Healing
25 Curzon Street
Basford
Newcastle-under-Lyme
Staffordshire ST5 0PD

**Faculty of Herbal Medicine
(General Council & Register of
Consultant Herbalists)**
Grosvenor House
40 Sea Way
Middleton-on-Sea
West Sussex PA22 7AA

**Osho School of Herbal Medicine and
Nature Care**
2 Bridge Farm Cottage
Station Road
Pulham Market
Near Diss
Norfolk IP21 3SJ
Tel: 0379 608201

**School of Phytotherapy (Herbal
Medicine)**
Bucksteep Manor
Bodle Street Green
Near Hailsham
East Sussex BN27 4RJ
Tel: 0323 833812/4

School of Planetary Herbalism
5 Turnpike Lane
Red Lodge
Bury Street
Edmunds
Suffolk IP28 8JZ
Tel: 0638 750140

HOMOEOPATHY

British Homoeopathic Association
27a Devonshire Street
London
W1N 1RJ

British Homoeopathy Research Group
101 Harley Street
London W1
Tel: 071 580 5489

British School of Homoeopathy
23 Sarum Avenue
Melksham
Wiltshire SN12 6BN
Tel: 0225 709687/790051

College of Classical Homoeopathy
Othergates Clinic
45 Barrington Street
Tiverton
Devon EX16 6QP
Tel: 0884 258143

College of Homoeopathy
Regents College
Inner Circle
Regents Park
London NW1 4NS
Tel: 071 487 7416

Faculty of Homoeopathy
Royal London Homeopathic Hospital
Great London Street
London WC1N 3HR
Tel: 071 837 8833 ext 85 or 72

Hahnemann College of Homoeopathy
243 The Broadway
Southall
Middlesex UB1 1NF
Tel: 081 574 4281

Hahnemann Society
Humane Education Centre
Avenue Lodge
Bounds Green Road
London N22 4EU
Tel: 081 889 1595

Healthways
3 Lorne Park Road
Bournemouth
Dorset BH1 1LD
Tel: 0202 28986

Homoeopathic Foundation
Marlborough House
Swanpool
Falmouth
Cornwall TR11 4HW

International Podiatric Association of Homoeopathic Medicine
141 Montrose Avenue
Edgware
Middlesex
Tel: 081 959 5421

London College of Classical Homoeopathy
At Morley College
61 Westminster Bridge Road
Waterloo
London SE1 7HT
Tel: 071 928 6199

National Association of Homoeopathic Groups
Alma Cottage
Brainsmead
Cuckfield
West Sussex RH17 5EY

North West College of Homoeopathy
23 Wilbraham Road
Fallowfield
Manchester M14 6FB
Tel: 061 257 2445/224 6809

Northern College of Homoeopathic Medicine
1st Floor
Swinburne House
Swinburne Street
Gateshead
Tyne and Wear NE8 1AX

Rugby School of Complementary Medicine
22 Bath Street
Rugby
Warwickshire CV21 3JF
Tel: 0788 62843

Scottish College of Homoeopathy
PO Box 33
Glasgow G2 2XG
Tel: 0360 311124

School of Homoeopathy
Misha Norland
Yondercott House
Uffculme
Devon EX15 3DR
Tel: 0884 40230

Society of Homoeopaths
2 Artizan Road
Northampton NN1 4HU
Tel: 0604 21400

UK Homoeopathic Medical Association
243 The Broadway
Southall
Middlesex UB1 3AN
Tel: 081 574 4281

HYPNOSIS AND HYPNOTHERAPY

**Academy of Hypnotherapy &
Professional Hypnotherapists Centre**
181 Cat Hill
Cockfosters
Hertfordshire EN4 8HS
Tel: 081 441 9685

**Association of Hypnotherapists in
Health Care**
Selly Oak Hospital
Birmingham

Association of Professional Therapists
55 The Spinney
Sidcup
Kent DA14 5NE
Tel: 081 300 7362

**Association of Qualified and Curative
Hypnotherapists**
10 Balaclava Road
Kings Heath
Birmingham B14 7SG
Tel: 021 444 5435

Association for Applied Hypnosis
55 Upgate
Louth
Lincolnshire LN11 9DH

British Hypnosis Research
Southpoint
8 Paston Place
Brighton BN2 1HA
Tel: 0273 693622

British Hypnotherapy Association
1 Wythburn Place
London W1H 5WL
Tel: 071 262 8852/723 4443

British Society of Hypnotherapists
37 Orbain Road
Fulham
London SW6 7JZ

**British Society of Medical and Dental
Hypnosis**
42 Links Road
Ashtead
Surrey KT21 2HJ
Tel 0372 273522

European Society of Medical Hypnosis
3 Troy Road
Morley
Leeds
West Yorkshire LS27 8JJ
Tel: 0532 533494

Federation of Hypnotherapists
10 Alexander Street
Bayswater
London W2 5NT
Tel: 071 727 2006

Hypnotherapy Centre Bournemouth
PO Box 180
Bournemouth BH8 8NH
Tel: 0202 396491

Hypnothink Foundation
PO Box 154
Cheltenham
Gloucestershire GL52 2SL

**Institute of Qualified Curative
Hypnotherapists**
91 St Ronans Road
Southsea
Hampshire PO4 0PR

**International Association of Hypno-
Analysts**
PO Box 80
Bournemouth
Dorset BH8 8NH
Tel: 0202 304626

**International Association of
Hypnotherapists**
1 Lowther Gardens
Bournemouth
Dorset BH8 8NH
Tel: 0202 304 624

International Institute of Hypnotists
c/o 95 Prospect Road
Woodford Green
Essex IG8 7ND
Tel: 081 505 8720

Midland Institute of Hypnotherapy
48 Hagley Road
Stourbridge
West Midlands DY8 1QH
Tel: 0384 371320

**National Association of
Hypnotherapists and Psychotherapists**
Ffynnonwen Natural Therapy Centre
Llangwyryfon
Aberystwyth
Dyfed
Tel: 09747 376

**National College of Hypnosis and
Psychotherapy**
12 Cross Street
Nelson
Lancashire BB9 7EN
Tel: 0282 699378

**National Council of Psychotherapists
and Hypnotherapy Register**
Stream Cottage
Wish Hill
Willingdon
East Sussex BN20 9HQ
Tel: 0323 501540

**National Register of Hypnotherapists
and Psychotherapists**
12 Cross Street
Nelson
Lancashire BB9 7EN
Tel: 0282 699378

Owl College of Hypnosis
2 Buchanan Street
Leigh
Greater Manchester WN7 1XT
Tel: 0942 677196

**Proudfoot School of Hypnosis &
Psychotherapy**
Belvedere Place
Scarborough
North Yorkshire YO11 2QX

**Register of Forensic and Investigative
Hypnosis**
42 Regent Street
Kingswood
Bristol
Avon BS15 2JS

**School of Hypnosis & Advanced
Psychotherapy**
23 Finsbury Park
London N4 2JX
Tel: 081 539 6991

**Society of Advanced Psychotherapy
Practitioners**
6 Mulberry Close
Mildenhall
Suffolk IP28 7LL
Tel: 0638 715581

Therapy Training College
8 & 10 Balaclava Street
Kings Heath
Birmingham B14 7SG
Tel: 021 444 5435

**UK Training College of
Hypnotherapy & Counselling**
10 Alexander Street
Bayswater
London W2 5NT
Tel: 071 221 1796/727 2006

World Federation of Hypnotherapists
Belmont Centre
46 Belmont Road
Ramsgate
Kent CT11 7QG
Tel: 0843 587929

IRIDOLOGY

Anglo-European School of Iridology
40 Stokewood Road
Bournemouth BH3 7NE
Tel: 0202 529793

British Register of Iridologists
PO Box 205
Cambridge CB3 7YF
Tel: 0654 51652

British School of Iridology
PO Box 205
Cambridge CB3 7YF
Tel: 0654 51652

College of Ophthalmic Somatology
24 Chapel Market
London N1 9EZ
Tel: 071 278 4610/1212

National Council and Register of Iridologists
Lacnunga
80 Portland Place
Bournemouth BH9 1NQ
Tel: 0202 529793

KINESIOLOGY

The Academy of Systematic Kinesiology
(Dept. CAM)
39 Browns Road
Surbiton
Surrey KT5 8ST
Tel: 081 399 3215

The Kinesiology School
8 Railey Mews
London NW5 2PA
Tel: 071 482 0698

MASSAGE

Academy of On-Site Massage
14 Brunswick Square
Hove BN3 1EH
Tel: 0273 720508

Adelaide School of Massage
24 Church Road
Hove
Sussex
Tel: 0273 732515

Allied School of Remedial Massage
37 Barnfield Close
Galmpton
Brixham
Devon TQ5 0LY
Tel: 0803 843492

Bournemouth School of Massage & Aromatherapy
14 Greenwood
Bournemouth BH9 2LH
Tel: 0202 513838

City and Guilds Institute
46 Britannia Street
London WC1X 9RG
Tel: 071 278 2468

Clare Maxwell-Hudson's Massage Training Centre
PO Box 457
London NW2 4ER
Tel: 081 450 6494

The Churchill Centre
22 Montagu Street
London W1H 1TB
Tel: 071 402 9475

College of Holistic Medicine
Sundrum Castle
Sundrum by Ayr KA6 5JY
Tel: 0292 709889

Essex School of Massage
Hadleigh Rise
Middle Street
Nazeing
Essex EN9 2LH

Gablescroft College of Natural Therapy
Church Street
Whittington
Oswestry
Shropshire SY11 4DT
Tel: 0691 659631

Gerda Boyesen Centre
Acacia House
Centre Avenue
Acton
London W3 7JX
Tel: 081 743 2437

International Therapy Examination Council (ITEC)
James House
Oakelbrook Mill
Newent
Gloucestershire GL18 1HD
Tel: 0531 821875

Leaves International School of Aromatherapy, Massage and Natural Therapy
Court Mills House
Court Street
Trowbridge
Wiltshire BA14 8BR

London College of Massage
5-6 Newman Passage
London W1
Tel: 071 978 8150/720 8817

London & Counties Society of Physiologists
100 Waterloo Road
Blackpool
Lancashire FY4 1A
Tel: 0253 403548

London School of Natural Health Sciences
32 Lodge Drive
Palmers Green
London N13 5JZ
Tel: 081 886 3120

London School of Sports Massage Ltd
88 Cambridge Street
London SW1V 4QG

Lyn Gorley School of Massage and Aromatherapy
The Vicarage
Church Road
Shaw
Newbury
Berkshire RG13 2DR
Tel: 0635 34365

Midlands School of Massage
The Castle Clinic
16 The Ropewalk
Nottingham NG1 7DT
Tel: 0602 472263

National School of Massage
72 Portland Street
Southport
Lancashire PR8 6QX

Neal Slack School of Massage
Stoneycrest
Kirtlington
Oxfordshire OX5 3HF
Tel: 0869 50420

Northern Institute of Massage
100 Waterloo Road
Blackpool
Lancashire FY4 1AW
Tel: 0253 403548

Oxford House Postgraduate Centre
2 Cheapside
Reading
Berkshire RG1 7AA
Tel: 0734 391361

Sara Thomas
15A Bridge Avenue
London W6

School of Physical Therapies
Lauriston House
London Road
Basingstoke
Hants RG21 2AA
Tel: 0256 475728

Shirley Goldstein
30 Gloucester Crescent
London NW1 7DL
Tel: 071 267 2552

'Touch for Health' Courses
42 Worthington Road
Surbiton
Surrey KT6 7RX

West London Schools of Therapeutic Massage,
Reflexology and Sports Therapy
41 St Luke's Road
London W11 1DD
Tel: 071 229 4672/7411

MEDITATION AND RELAXATION

Audio Ltd
26 Wendell Road
London W12 9RT
Tel: 081 743 1518

Centre for Autogenic Training
101 Harley Street
London W1N 1DF
Tel: 071 935 1811

Relaxation for Living
29 Burwood Park Road
Walton on Thames
Surrey KT12 5LH

Salisbury Centre
2 Salisbury Road
Edinburgh
Lothian
Scotland EH16 5AB

School of Meditation
158 Holland Park Avenue
London W11 4UH
Tel: 071 603 6116

London Sufi Centre
21 Lancaster Road
London W11 1QL
Tel: 071 229 1064/221 3215

Transcendental Meditation
Mentmore
Leighton Buzzard
Bedfordshire LU7 0QH

Yoga for Health Foundation
Ickwell Bury
Ickwell Green
Northill
Biggleswade
Bedfordshire
Tel: 076727 271

NATUROPATHY

British College of Naturopathy & Osteopathy
Frazer House
6 Netherhall Gardens
London NW3 5RR
Tel: 071 435 7830

British Natural Hygiene Society
Shalimar
3 Harold Grove
Frinton-on-Sea
Essex CO13 9BD
Tel: 0255 672823

British Naturopathic and Osteopathic Association
Frazer House
6 Netherhall Gardens
London NW3 5RR
Tel: 071 435 8728

College of Osteopathic Practitioners' Association (Incorporating Naturopaths)
110 Thorkhill Road
Thames Ditton
Surrey KT7 0UW
Tel: 081 398 3308

General Council and Register of Naturopaths
Frazer House
6 Netherhall Gardens
London NW3 5RR
Tel: 071 435 8728

Incorporated Society British Naturopaths
Kingston
The Coach House
293 Gilmerton Road
Edinburgh EH16 5UQ
Tel: 031 664 3435

Natural Therapeutic and Osteopathic Society and Register
14 Marford Road
Wheathampstead
Hertfordshire AL4 8AS
Tel: 058283 3950

Osteopathic and Naturopathic Guild
Marlborough House
Swanpool
Falmouth
Cornwall TR11 4HW
Tel: 0326 317321

NURSING AND COMPLEMENTARY THERAPIES

The Didsbury Trust
Sherbourne Cottage
Litton
Near Bath
Avon BA3 4PS
Tel: 0761 241640
(A registered charity dedicated to the care, support and education of nurses and health care professionals through the promotion of the healing arts)

'Holistic Nurses' School of Nursing
Royal Free Hospital
Pond Street
Hampstead
London NW3 2QG
Tel: 071 794 0550 ext 3733

Complementary Therapies in Nursing Special Interest Group
The Royal College of Nursing (RCN)
20 Cavendish Square
London W1M 0AB
Tel 071 409 3333
(Contact: Paul Denton)

OSTEOPATHY

British College of Naturopathy and Osteopathy
Frazer House
6 Netherhall Gardens
London NW3 5RR
Tel: 071 435 7830/6464

British and European Osteopathic Association
6 Adelaide Road
Teddington
Middlesex TW11 0AY
Tel: 081 977 8532

British Naturopathic and Osteopathic
Association
Frazer House
6 Netherhall Gardens
London NW3 5RR
Tel: 071 435 8728

British Osteopathic Association
8-10 Boston Place
London NW1 6QH
Tel: 262 5250/1128

British School of Osteopathy
1-4 Suffolk St
London SW1Y 4HG
Tel: 071 930 9254

College of Osteopaths Educational
Trust
1 Furzehill Road
Borehamwood
Hertfordshire WD6 2DG
Tel: 081 905 1937

College of Osteopaths Practitioners
Association
(Incorporating Naturopaths)
110 Thorkhill Road
Thames Ditton
Surrey KT7 0UW
Tel: 081 398 3308

Cranial Osteopathic Association
478 Baker Street
Enfield
Middlesex EN1 3QS
Tel: 081 367 5561

European School of Osteopathy
104 Tonbridge Road
Maidstone
Kent ME16 8SL
Tel: 0622 671558

Faculty of Osteopathy
PO Box 43
Lytham St Annes
Lancashire FY8 1PT

General Council and Register of
Osteopaths
56 London Street
Reading
Berkshire TH1 4SQ
Tel: 0734 576589

Guild of Osteopaths (London)
59 Connaught Avenue
Shoreham
West Sussex BN4 5WL

London School of Osteopathy
Whitelands College
West Hill
London SW15 3SN
Tel: 081 785 2267

Maidstone College of Osteopathy
30 Tonbridge Road
Maidstone
Kent ME16 8RT
Tel: 0622 752375

Natural Therapeutic and Osteopathic
Society and Register
14 Marford Road
Wheathampstead
Hertfordshire AL4 8AS
Tel: 058283 3950

Osteopathic Association of Great
Britain
62 Messina Avenue
London NW6 4LE
Tel: 071 372 3206

Osteopathic and Naturopathic Guild
Marlborough House
Swanpool
Falmouth
Cornwall TR11 4HW
Tel: 0326 317321

Oxford School of Osteopathy
Doyle Croft
PO Box 67
Banbury
Oxfordshire OX16 8LE
Tel: 0869 35383

Society of Osteopaths
62 Bower Mount Road
Maidstone
Kent
Tel: 0622 674656

PSYCHOTHERAPY

Arbours Association
6 Church Lane
London N8 7BU
Tel: 081 340 7646

Association of Humanistic Psychology Practitioners (AHPP)
45 Litchfield Way
London NW11 6NU
Tel: 081 455 8737

Association for Group and Individual Psychotherapy
1 Fairbridge Road
London N19 3EN
Tel: 071 272 7013

Association for Humanistic Psychology in Great Britain
26 Huddlestone Road
London E7 0AN
Tel: 081 555 3077

Association of Child Psychotherapists
Burgh House
New End Square
London NW3 1LT
Tel: 071 794 8881

British Association for Counselling
37a Sheep Street
Rugby
Warwickshire CV21 3BX
Tel: 0788 78328/9

British Association of Psychotherapists
121 Hendon Lane
London N3 3PR
Tel: 081 346 1747

British Psycho-Analytical Society
63 New Cavendish Street
London W1
Tel: 071 580 4952

Centre for Counselling and Psychotherapy Education
21 Lancaster Road
London W11 1QL
Tel: 071 221 3215

Chiron Centre for Holistic Psychotherapy
26 Eaton Rise
Ealing
London W5 2ER
Tel: 081 997 5219

College of Psychotherapeutics
White Lodge
Stockland Green Road
Speldhurst
Tunbridge Wells
Kent TN3 0TT
Tel: 0892 863166

Gestalt Centre
64 Warwick Road
St Albans
Hertfordshire AL1 4DL
Tel: 0727 64806

Holistic Rebirthing Institute
18a Great Percy Street
London WC1X 0QP
Tel: 071 833 0741

Institute of Psychiatry
De Crespigny Park
London SE5
Tel: 071 703 5411

Institute of Psychosynthesis
The Barn
Nan Clark's Lane
Mill Hill
London NW7 4HH
Tel: 081 959 2330

Institute of Transactional Analysis
BM Box 4104
London WC1N 3XX
Tel: 071 404 5011

Minster Centre
55 Minster Road
London NW2
Tel: 071 435 9200

National College of Hypnosis and Psychotherapy
12 Cross Street
Nelson
Lancashire BB0 7EN
Tel: 0262 699378

Proudfoot School of Hypnosis and Psychotherapy
Belvedere Place
Scarborough
North Yorkshire YO11 2QX
Tel: 0723 363638

School of Hypnosis and Advanced Psychotherapy
28 Finsbury Park Road
London N4 2JX
Tel: 081 539 6991

Sheffield School of Christian Psychotherapy and Counselling
512 Fulwood Road
Sheffield
South Yorkshire S10 3QD
Tel: 0742 307073

West Midlands Bioenergetic Group
c/o West Mount House
146a Eastern Road
Brighton
East Sussex BN2 2AE
Tel: 0273 697732

Westminster Pastoral Foundation
23 Kensington Square
London W8 5HN
Tel: 071 937 6956

RADIONICS

British Society of Dowsers
Sycamore Cottage
Tamley Lane
Hastingleigh
Ashford
Kent TN25 5HW
Tel: 023375 253

College of Radionic Science and Natural Therapeutics
B C M Florin
London WC1N 3XX

Confederation of Radionic and Radiesthetic Organisations
c/o Maperton Trust
Wincanton
Somerset BA9 8EM
Tel: 0963 32651

Delawarr Society of Radionics
Delawarr Laboratories
Raleigh Park Road
Oxford OX2 9BB
Tel: 0865 248572

Enermed Institute of Radionics and Radiesthesia
4a the Parade
Station Road
Sturminster
Newton
Dorset DT10 1BA
Tel: 0258 73986

International Federation of Radionics
c/o 21 Portland Place
London W1N 3AF
Tel: 071 636 9543

Keith Mason School of Radionics
21 Portland Place
London W1N 3AF
Tel: 071 636 9543

Orly Institute
6 Pembroke Avenue
Hove
West Sussex BN3 5DA
Tel: 0273 732519

Psionic Medical Society
Garden Cottage
Beacon Hill Park
Hindhead
Surrey GU26 6HU
Tel: 042873 5752

Radionic Association
Baerlein House
Goose Green
Deddington
Oxford OX5 4SZ
Tel: 0869 38852

School of Radionics
45 Silbridge Rise
Sturminster Newton
Dorset DT10 1BP
Tel: 0258 72784

Sensonics Association
18a Church Street
Oswestry
Shropshire SY11 3SP
Tel: 0691 670104

Phoenix College of Radionics
62 Alexandra Road
Hemel Hempstead
Hertfordshire HP2 4AQ
Tel: 0442 243333

REFLEXOLOGY

Association of Chartered Physiotherapists with an Interest in Reflex Zone Therapy ACPIRT
Membership is open to physiotherapists, nurses, midwives and occupational therapists.
Secretary: Mrs Susan Hollenberry, MCSP, 7 Waggon Road
Hadley Wood
Hertfordshire EN4 0PW
(Please enclose s.a.e.)

Association of Reflexologists
27 Old Gloucester Street
London WC1N 3XX
Tel: 081 445 0154

Bayly School of Reflexology
Monks Orchard
Whitbourne
Worcestershire WR6 5RB
Tel: 0886 21207

British Reflexology Association
Monks Orchard
Whitbourne
Worcestershire WR6 5RB
Tel: 0886 21207

British School - Reflex Zone Therapy of the Feet
87 Oakington Avenue
Wembley Park
Middlesex HA9 8HY
Tel: 081 908 2201

British School of Reflexology
Holistic Healing Centre
92 Sheering Road
Old Harlow
Essex CM17 0JW

Chiltern Institute of Reflexology
23 Poplars Road
Buckingham
Buckinghamshire MK18 1BQ
Tel: 0280 813658

Churchill Centre
22 Montague Street
London W1H 1TB
Tel: 071 402 9475

College of Reflexology
50 Sydney Die Court
Sporle
Kings Lynn
Norfolk PE32 2EE
Tel: 0760 725437

Crane School of Reflexology
135 Collins Meadow
Harlow
Essex CM19 4EJ
Tel: 0279 21682

Dallamore College of Advanced Reflexology
50 Sydney Dye Court
Sporle
Kings Lynn
Norfolk PE32 2EE
Tel: 0760 725437

Dilworth School of Reflexology
193 Tring Road
Aylesbury
Buckinghamshire HP20 1JH
Tel: 0296 24854

Gablecroft College of Natural Therapy
Church Street
Whittington
Shropshire
Tel: 0691 659631

International Institute of Reflexology
Administration Office
28 Hollyfield Avenue
London N11 3BY
Tel: 081 368 0865

Janice Ellicot School of Reflexology
42 Alder Lodge
Stevenage Road
London SW6 6NP
Tel: 071 386 9914

Mary Martin School of Reflexology
37 Standale Grove
Ruislip
Middlesex HA4 7UA
Tel: 0895 635 621

Metamorphic Association
67 Ritherdon Road
Tooting
London SW17 8QE
Tel: 081 672 5951

Midland School of Reflextherapy
5 Church Street
Warwick
Warwickshire CV34 4AB
Tel: 0926 491071

Moorlands Natural Medicine Teaching Centre
24 South Road
Newton Abbot
Devon TQ12 1HQ
Tel: 0626 65493

Oxford House Postgraduate Centre
2 Cheapside
Reading
Berkshire RG1 7AA
Tel: 0734 391361

Raworth Centre
Smallburgh
Beare Green
Dorking
Surrey RH5 4QA
Tel: 0306 712623

Reflexology Centre
8 Russell Court
London Lane
Bromley
Kent BR1 4HX

School of Physical Therapies
Lauriston House
London Road
Basingstoke
Hampshire RG21 2AA
Tel: 0256 475728

Scottish School of Reflexology
2 Wheatfield Road
Ayr KA7 2XB
Tel: 0292 280494

West London School of Foot Reflex Therapy
41 St Luke's Road
London W11 1DD
Tel: 071 474 7212

West London School of Therapeutic Massage & Reflexology
41a St Luke's Road
London W11 1DD
Tel: 071 229 7411/4672

SHIATSU

See Acupressure and Shiatsu

TRADITIONAL MEDICINE

Eagles Wing (Teachings of the Medicine Wheel)
58 Westbere Road
London NW2 3RU
Tel: 071 435 8174

International Society of Ayurveda
(Traditional Indian Medical Science)
7 Ravenscroft Avenue
London NW11 0SA

Tibet Foundation
43 New Oxford Street
London WC1A 1BH
Tel: 071 379 0634

YOGA

British School of Yoga
46 Hagley Road
Stourbridge
West Midlands DY8 1QD
Tel: 0384 371320

British Wheel of Yoga
1 Hamilton Place
Boston Road
Sleaford
Lincolnshire NG34 7ES
Tel: 0529 306851

Centre for Yoga Studies
PO Box 158
Bath BA1 2YG
Tel: 0225 26327

Chinese Yoga Federation
Kongoryuji Temple
East Dergham
Norfolk NR19 1AS
Tel: 0362 693962

Iyengar Yoga Institute
223a Randolph Avenue
London W9 1NL
Tel: 071 624 3080

Kundalini Yoga Foundation
61 Sladedale Road
London SE18 1PY
Tel: 081 854 8748

London Centre for Yoga and Shiatsu
49b Onslow Gardens
London N10 3JY
Tel: 081 444 0103

Yoga Biomedical Trust
PO Box 140
Cambridge CB1 1PU
Tel: 0223 67301/27747

Yoga for Health Foundation
Ickwell Bury
Northill
Biggleswade
Bedfordshire
Tel: 076727 271

Section 5:
Choosing a Complementary Therapies Course

The following information was supplied by the Royal College of Nursing, Department of Nursing Policy and Practice Complementary Therapies in Nursing Special Interest Group.

CHOOSING A COURSE

The following checklist may be helpful for nurses interested in choosing a complementary therapies course:

* what qualifications are needed?

* how long is the course?

* what will it cost and will your employer help fund it?

* is there scope for using the therapy in your area of work?

* is there an aptitude test or can anyone join the course who can pay the fees?

When looking at course content and structure it is worth considering:

* is the course validated by any examining bodies?

* what European Community regulations affect the therapy in question?

* is there accreditation, supervised practice, a practical, theory, anatomy, physiology or pathology examination; are counselling and communication skills included, does the course use a holistic approach, what are the qualifications of the teaching staff, what is the teacher/pupil ratio, does the course offer business skills?

Talk to other nurses and find out their evaluation of the course you are considering. See if there is a taster weekend at which you can get the feel of the course before parting with fees.

Section 6:
Acknowledgements

The Publishers and Editors are immensely grateful to the following people for their help and advice in preparing this Appendix: firstly to Hazel Bently, Publisher, *International Journal of Alternative & Complementary Medicine* for so kindly sending a copy of the *1990 Natural Medicine Practitioners Yearbook*, which proved invaluable; and to the Royal College of Nursing, for so kindly allowing us to reproduce Section 5 of the Appendix, and especially to Paul Denton, RCN Adviser in Research, for his advice more generally.

RECOMMENDED FURTHER READING

- *1993 Natural Medicine Practitioners Yearbook*: A complete quick reference guide to more than 2000 sources of benefit to the health care professional in Britain.
Published by Reasonhold Limited, publishers of the *International Journal of Alternative & Complementary Medicine*, Green Library, Homewood NHS Trust (DQH), Guildford Road, Chertsey, Surrey KT16 OQA. Tel: 0932 874333. Subscriptions: 0276 451527.

- Maher, G. *Start a Career in Complementary Medicine*: A Manual/Directory of Courses in Alternative and Complementary Medicine. Second Edition 1992, Tackmart Publishing, P.O. Box 140, Harrow, Middlesex HA3 OUY.

Index